FOOD SELECTION AND PREPARATION

A Laboratory Manual

Frank D. Conforti
Iowa State University Press, Ames

Frank D. Conforti, Ph.D., is Associate Professor of Human Nutrition, Foods, and Exercise in the Foods Department, Virginia Tech, Blacksburg. He also has extensive commercial experience in the food industry as Director of Quality Control, Borden's, and Director of Quality Assurance, American Foods Laboratory. Dr. Conforti's research interests are in the interaction of ingredients and their effect on quality in a food system, particularly the baking quality of fat substitutes.

Orders: 1-800-862-6657
Office: 1-515-292-0140
Fax: 1-515-292-3348
Web site: www.isupress.edu

♾ Printed on acid-free paper in the United States of America

First edition, 1997

International Standard Book Number: 0-8138-2714-0

Last digit is the print number: 9 8 7 6 5 4 3

CONTENTS

PREFACE

My objective in writing this manual for a foods laboratory setting was to create a learning tool for the student in food service, hospitality management, dietetics, or family and consumer science education. The 1990's has witnessed a shift to a more healthy approach to eating. American consumers are starting to make new choices in their diets.

The student should learn how to prepare nutritious food and how to make substitutions when necessary, yet still maintain the integrity and quality of food. Before this can be accomplished, the student must learn the preliminaries in food preparation. It is important to understand the function of an ingredient in a food system. Once this is mastered, the proper selection and manipulation can be made for a specific recipe. The quality and acceptability of the food should be paramount to the student, and emphasis must be placed on understanding and following a recipe to produce an acceptable end-product.

This manual has been set up so that the student will gain a deeper understanding of the various food preparation principles by carrying out the exercises and preparing the recipes. Vocabulary words are listed and questions are raised to aid in understanding the basic concepts of each unit. Recipes are also included to enlighten the learning experience and to give a more "hands-on" approach to reinforce the concepts presented in lectures. Some recipes have been adapted to meet the new eating trends. Traditional recipes (yellow cake, white sauce, pie crust, etc.) are included so the student can learn proper preparation techniques and ingredient functionality and can understand the mechanism involved in a particular food system in order to make the proper substitution when the need arises.

Each laboratory is an independent unit and can be assigned according to any sequence chosen by the instructor. There are a number of recipes in each unit, but they all do not have to be included in the lesson, especially if some laboratory periods run for 2 hours instead of 3 hours. A careful selection of activities by the instructor should give the student a firm basis in foods and a clear understanding of the proper selection and manipulation of ingredients that will lead to quality preparation.

I hope you will enjoy this manual. Not only will it provide a door to the spectrum of foods, it will bring a deeper appreciation of and respect for food preparation. If you keep this manual as a reference after completing this course, it will continue to be a source of information for solving the most common problems that arise in food selection and preparation.

ACKNOWLEDGMENTS

I would like to express my appreciation to the following people who have contributed to the manual: Marilynn Schnepf, University of Nebraska, whose influence served as a basis for this manual; Eleanor Schlenker and Janet M. Johnson, Virginia Polytechnic Institute and State University, whose enthusiastic support led to the publication of the manual; Sherry Saville, Virginia Polytechnic Institute and State University, whose countless hours and expertise at the computer helped to get the manuscript into book form; and the students whose suggestions and participation over the years have made this manual a reality for others to appreciate. The input of these people has been invaluable and has helped to make this manual unique.

LABORATORY 1

Measuring Techniques

LABORATORY 1
MEASURING TECHNIQUES

Proper measuring techniques must be emphasized to ensure success in food preparation. There are differences when measuring liquid and dry ingredients, and the student must learn these techniques as soon as possible. This laboratory exercise will introduce the student to the proper techniques in measuring.

VOCABULARY

boiling point	opaque	solute
meniscus	simmering	solvent

MEASURING TECHNIQUES

The American Standards Association has defined the capacities of various measures, but not all measuring equipment has been standardized to meet these specifications. Variations of 5%, more or less than the standard, are allowable.

NONMETRIC MEASURES OF VOLUME

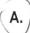

A. DRY MEASURES

A set of fractional measuring cups includes measures for 1/4 cup, 1/3 cup, 1/2 cup, and 1 cup. These measures are used for dry ingredients and solid fats. Ingredients vary in the way they pack down, lump, or cling to the measuring cup. Use the following guidelines when measuring:

1. All-purpose flour, cake flour, granulated sugar, and confectioner's sugar should be lightly spooned into the appropriate size dry measuring cup. **Do not shake or pat down**. Use a straight-edge spatula or knife to level off ingredients (*FIG.1*).

> *FIG.1*: Spoon dry ingredients lightly into cup and level off with a straight-edge spatula. (Reprinted with permission from Helen Charley, *Food Study Manual*, Ronald Press, NY.)

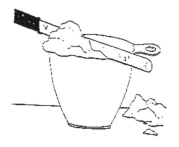

2. Nuts, coconut, and bread crumbs should be spooned into the cup and packed down lightly.
3. Brown sugar should be spooned into the dry measure cup and packed down firmly with spatula or spoon.
4. Solid fats include hydrogenated shortening, lard, margarine, and butter. The solid fat should be packed into the dry measure with firm pressure.

B. SMALL AMOUNTS OF INGREDIENTS

1. Baking powder, baking soda, salt, and spices are used in such small amounts that they must be measured in small capacity measures of 1 tablespoon or less.
2. Ingredients should be stirred and free of lumps.
3. The desired measure is dipped into the ingredient and leveled off.
4. Usually the measuring spoons are found as 1/4 teaspoon (tsp.), 1/2 teaspoon, 1 teaspoon, and 1 tablespoon (tbsp.).

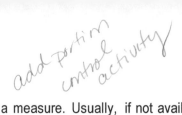

5. Some measuring spoon sets are available that contain 1/8 teaspoon as a measure. Usually, if not available and if less than 1/4 teaspoon is needed, this measure can be filled, leveled, and half or more of its contents removed.

C. LIQUIDS

1. Oil, honey, milk, molasses, juices, water, melted fat, and other liquid ingredients should be measured in a graduated, transparent liquid measure with a pour spout.
2. Fill the measure to the desired graduation and check it by holding the measure at eye level so that the bottom of the meniscus - the curved, upper surface of the liquid - matches the desired line on the side of the measure (*FIG.2*).
3. Opaque liquids that do not show a meniscus are measured by aligning the top of the liquid with the line on the measure.
4. Many liquids, especially oil and honey, tend to cling to the sides of the cup. To obtain an accurate transfer of the liquid, it is essential that the inside of the cup be scraped out with a rubber spatula.

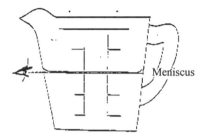

FIG.2: Read the measure by holding it at eye level so the bottom of the meniscus matches the desired line on the side of the measure. (Reprinted with permission from Helen Charley, *Food Study Manual*, Ronald Press, NY.)

D. OTHER MEASURING ADVICE

1. If the recipe specifies 3 teaspoons of baking powder, a tablespoon should be used to make the measurement. To measure 3 separate teaspoons introduces greater chance of error in measurement.
2. When the recipe specifies less than 1 cup of liquid, such as milk, and the measurement is made in a 2 cup graduated measure, there is also greater chance of error.
3. It is important to use the measuring utensil that is closest in size to the amount of the ingredient for greater accuracy.

EQUIVALENT MEASURES:

1 tablespoon	= 3 teaspoons		3/4 cup	= 12 tablespoons
1/8 cup	= 2 tablespoons		1 cup	= 16 tablespoons or 1/2 pint
1/4 cup	= 4 tablespoons		1 pint	= 2 cups
1/3 cup	= 5 tablespoons + 1 teaspoon		1 quart	= 4 cups or 2 pints
1/2 cup	= 8 tablespoons		1 gallon	= 4 quarts
2/3 cup	= 10 tablespoon + 2 teaspoons			

I. TO LEARN CORRECT TECHNIQUES FOR MEASURING INGREDIENTS

A. FLOUR (All-Purpose or Cake Flour)

1. **Method 1**

   a. Fill 1/2 cup dry measure by dipping into can of flour.
   b. Level with spatula.
   c. Weigh flour on a gram scale and record weight in the table.
   d. Repeat.

2. **Method 2**

    a.   Place a 1/2 cup dry measure on a piece of waxed paper 12 inches square.
    b.   Sift flour directly into a cup until cup overflows. Do not let sifter touch the cup.
    c.   Level flour with the edge of a spatula.
    d.   Weigh flour and record weight in the table.
    e.   Repeat.

3. **Method 3**

    a.   Stir flour in canister to lighten.
    b.   Carefully spoon flour 1 tablespoon at a time into 1/2 cup dry measure.
    c.   Level flour with the edge of a spatula.
    d.   Weigh flour and record weight in the table.
    e.   Repeat.

TABLE FOR EVALUATION OF THE WEIGHT OF 1/2 CUP OF FLOUR			
Method	Trial 1	Trial 2	Standard Weight*
1	2.5 oz	2.5 oz	
2	2.0 oz	2.0 oz	
3	1.9 oz	1.9 oz	

*All purpose: 1/2 cup sifted: 58.0 g; 1/2 cup unsifted, spooned: 62.5 g.
*Cake flour: 1/2 cup, sifted: 48 g; 1/2 cup spooned: 55.5 g.
Source: *Handbook of Food Preparation: Food and Nutrition Section*, 9th Edition, 1993, American Home Economics Association, p. 182.

QUESTIONS

1.   Which method of measuring flour yields the best check? Why?

2.   What would cause a difference in the weight from the standard?

3.   How would you substitute all-purpose flour for cake flour in a recipe?

B.) **SUGAR: GRANULATED AND BROWN**

1. **Method 1**

    a.   Fill a 1/4 cup dry measure with granulated sugar by dipping it into sugar can.
    b.   Level the sugar with the edge of the spatula.
    c.   Weigh sugar and record in the table.
    d.   Repeat.

2.   **Method 2**

   a.   Fill a 1/4 cup dry measure with brown sugar by spooning sugar into cup.
   b.   Level the sugar with the edge of the spatula.
   c.   Weigh sugar and record in the table.
   d.   Repeat.

3.   **Method 3**

   a.   Fill a 1/4 cup dry measure with brown sugar by pressing sugar into the measuring cup.
   b.   Level the sugar with the edge of the spatula.
   c.   Weigh sugar and record in the table.
   d.   Repeat.

TABLE FOR EVALUATION OF THE WEIGHT OF 1/4 CUP OF SUGAR			
Method	Trial 1	Trial 2	Standard Weight
1	2g 1.75	1.75	
2	1 1/2 .	1.5	
3	2.0g	2.0	

*Light brown sugar, packed: 1/4 cup = 50 g. Dark brown sugar, packed: 1/4 cup = 50 g. Granulated sugar: 1/4 cup = 50 g.
Source: *Handbook of Food Preparation: Food and Nutrition Section*, 9th Edition, 1993, American Home Economics Association, p. 195.

QUESTION

1.   How does the method for measuring brown sugar differ from that of measuring granulated sugar?

C. LIQUID

1.   **Method 1**

   a.   Fill a liquid measuring cup with water to 1/2 cup mark.
   b.   Place cup on a level surface and position yourself at eye level with the water before attempting to read the water level (*FIG.2*).
   c.   Transfer all the water from the measuring cup to a 100 ml graduated cylinder and read the volume in milliliters.
   d.   Record the volume in the table and repeat.
   e.   Repeat steps a through d, but use milk.

2.   **Method 2**

   a.   Fill a 1/4 cup dry measure with water.
   b.   Place measure upon a level surface and position yourself at eye level with the water before reading the water level.
   c.   Transfer all the water from the cup to a 100 ml graduated cylinder and read the volume in milliliters.
   d.   Record the volume in the table and repeat.

5

TABLE FOR EVALUATION OF LIQUID MEASUREMENTS			
Method of Measurement	Trial 1	Trial 2	Standard Volume*
1			
2			

*1 cup liquid measure = 236 ml; 1/4 cup liquid measure = 59 ml.
Source: *Handbook of Food Preparation: Food and Nutrition Section*, 9th Edition, 1993, American Home Economics Association, p. 180.

QUESTIONS

1. Was there a difference in measurement between the two liquids and why?

2. Would you recommend liquid measure or dry measure? Both? Why?

3. List some reasons why your method of measurement might differ from the standard.

D. FATS

1. Method 1

a. Fill a 1/4 cup dry measure with a hydrogenated fat.
b. Use a rubber spatula and press fat into cup making sure there are no air pockets.
c. Level off with a spatula.
d. Carefully remove fat from cup with a rubber spatula and weigh.
e. Record weight in the table and repeat.

2. Method 2

a. Melt hydrogenated fat in a saucepan over **low heat**.
b. Take 1 cup liquid measuring cup and pour melted fat up to the 1/4 cup measure mark.
c. Weigh and record the weight in the table. Repeat.

TABLE FOR EVALUATION OF THE WEIGHT OF 1/4 CUP HYDROGENATED FAT			
Method	Trial 1	Trial 2	Standard Measure*
1	1.25 oz	N/a	
2	1.0 oz	n/a	

*Hydrogenated shortening, solid, 1/4 cup = 46 g.
Source: *Handbook of Food Preparation: Food and Nutrition Section*, 9th Edition, 1993, American Home Economics Association, p. 175.

QUESTIONS

1.   What precautions should you take for measuring fats?

2.   Account for the differences in weight of the fats.

II.   WATER AND THERMOMETRY

1.   Most of the changes brought about in foods by cooking take place in a watery medium.
2.   Water absorbs heat from the hot unit through the cooking utensil and transfers this heat to the food.
3.   Water sets its limit to how hot it gets, while fat can go to higher extremities.
4.   The intensity of the heat is measured by a thermometer (either in °F or °C).

A.   FACTS ON USING A THERMOMETER

1.   The bulb must be completely covered with hot liquid.
2.   The bulb should not touch the sides or bottom of the utensil.
3.   There are 100° between the boiling point and the freezing point of water on the centigrade scale.
4.   There are 180° between the boiling point and the freezing point of water on the Fahrenheit scale.
5.   Therefore:
    a. $1°C = 1.8°F$
    b. $°C = (°F - 32) \div 1.8$
    c. $°F = (°C \times 1.8) + 32$

B.   LEARN TO RECOGNIZE COMMONLY USED TEMPERATURES

Heat water to each temperature specified in the table and feel or note its appearance.

TABLE FOR EVALUATION OF COMMONLY USED TEMPERATURES			
	Description	Temperature	
		°F	°C
Room		77.0	25
Lukewarm		98.6	37
Scalding*		149.0	65
Simmering		185.0	85
Boiling Slowly		212.0	100
Boiling Rapidly		212.0	100

*The temperature varies with material being scalded.

QUESTIONS

1.   Explain what happens when water boils.

2. Name some instances when scalding temperature is used in food preparation.

3. What would happen if salt was added to boiling water? If sugar was added?

C. DETERMINING THE ACCURACY OF LABORATORY OVENS

1. Take an oven thermometer and calibrate your ovens. Place rack in the middle position of the oven. Use 350°F as a standard to go by.
2. Record oven temperature: _____.

QUESTIONS

1. Why is it important that the temperature of the oven be exact?

2. In what positions would you place the oven rack if you cooked:

    a. a single loaf of bread?

    b. two layer cake?

    c. a tube cake?

    d. a standing rib roast?

III. APPLICATION OF MEASURING TECHNIQUES: COOKIES

OBJECTIVE

1. To practice proper measuring techniques involving dry and liquid measures.
2. To familiarize the student with reading and following a recipe.

A. CHOCOLATE CHIP COOKIES

1/3 cup shortening   3/4 cup all-purpose flour
1/4 cup sugar   1/4 teaspoon baking soda
1/4 cup brown sugar   1/4 teaspoon salt
1 small egg   3 ounces chocolate chips
1/4 teaspoon vanilla extract

1. Preheat oven to 375˚F. Make sure oven rack is in the middle position.
2. Cream shortening, sugar, brown sugar, egg, and vanilla.
3. Sift together flour, soda, and salt; mix with sugar mixture. Stir in chocolate chips.
4. Drop by rounded teaspoonfuls about 2 inches apart on ungreased baking sheet.
5. Bake for 8-10 minutes. When edges start to brown slightly, remove from oven.
6. Remove cookies to cooling rack with wide spatula.

B. CHOCOLATE CHIP COOKIES (LOW FAT VARIATION)

1/2 cup granulated sugar minus 1 tablespoon
1/4 cup light brown sugar, packed
1/4 cup margarine, softened
1 teaspoon vanilla
1 egg white

1 cup + 1 tablespoon all-purpose flour
1/2 teaspoon baking soda
1/4 teaspoon salt
1/2 cup miniature semisweet chocolate chips

1. Heat oven to 375˚F.
2. Mix sugars, margarine, vanilla, and egg white in large bowl.
3. Stir in flour, baking soda, and salt.
4. Stir in chocolate chips.
5. Drop by rounded teaspoonfuls about 2 inches apart on ungreased baking sheet.
6. Bake for 8-10 minutes or until golden brown.
7. Cool slightly; remove from cookie sheet.

C. OATMEAL COOKIES (BASIC RECIPE)

1/2 cup all-purpose flour
1/2 teaspoon baking powder
1/4 teaspoon salt
1/2 teaspoon cinnamon
1/4 cup + 2 tablespoons milk
1/4 cup + 2 tablespoons shortening

1/2 cup light brown sugar
1 egg
1 1/2 cups quick cooking oatmeal
1/4 cup chopped walnuts
1/4 cup coconut

1. Preheat oven to 375˚F. Make sure oven rack is in the middle position.
2. Sift together flour, baking powder, salt, and cinnamon into a bowl.
3. Add shortening, sugar, egg, and half the milk. Beat until smooth.
4. Add the balance of the milk and oatmeal. Mix thoroughly.
5. Add walnuts and coconut.
6. Drop from a teaspoon onto a greased cookie sheet.
7. Bake 12-15 minutes. When cookies are dry and edges start to brown, remove from oven.
8. Remove cookies from cookie sheet to cooling rack.

D. OATMEAL SPICE COOKIES (LOW FAT VERSION)

2 1/4 cups quick-cooking oats
2 tablespoons orange juice
1 cup all-purpose flour
1/2 teaspoon baking soda
1/2 teaspoon baking powder
1/4 teaspoon salt
1/4 teaspoon cinnamon
1/8 teaspoon cloves

1/8 teaspoon nutmeg
3 tablespoons margarine
3 tablespoons canola oil
1 cup packed dark brown sugar
1 tablespoon molasses
1 large egg white
2 teaspoons vanilla extract
About 2 teaspoons granulated sugar, for shaping cookies

1. Preheat oven to 350˚F. Spray several baking sheets with PAM and set aside.

9

2. Stir together oats and juice in a medium-sized bowl; set aside.
3. Thoroughly stir together flour, baking soda, baking powder, salt, cinnamon, cloves, and nutmeg in a medium-sized bowl; set aside.
4. In a large mixing bowl, with mixer set at medium speed, beat margarine and oil until well blended and smooth.
5. Add brown sugar, molasses, egg white, and vanilla and beat until fluffy and smooth.
6. Beat in flour mixture.
7. Using a large wooden spoon, stir in oat mixture until thoroughly incorporated.
8. Shape dough into 1-inch balls, and place 3 inches apart on baking sheets. Flatten cookies using the bottom of a glass that has been lightly greased and dipped in the 2 tablespoons of sugar. Dip the glass in sugar after flattening each cookie.
9. Bake cookies for 8-10 minutes.
10. Let stand on sheets for 3-4 minutes. Using a spatula, transfer cookies to racks and let stand until completely cooled.

E. BROWNIES

2 ounces unsweetened chocolate	1/2 teaspoon vanilla
1/3 cup shortening	1/2 cup + 2 tablespoons all-purpose flour
1 cup sugar	1/2 teaspoon salt
3/4 teaspoon instant coffee granules	1/2 cup chocolate chips
2 eggs	1/2 cup nuts, chopped

1. Preheat oven to 350°F. Make sure rack is in the middle position.
2. Grease an $8 \times 8 \times 2$ inch square pan.
3. Melt chocolate and shortening in a 2 quart saucepan over **low heat**.
4. Remove from heat and mix in the sugar, eggs, instant coffee granules, and vanilla.
5. Stir in the remaining ingredients. Spread in pan.
6. Bake 30 minutes or until the brownies start to pull away from the sides of the pan. **Do not overbake**.
7. Cool slightly. Cut into bars, about $2 \times 1 1/2$ inches. Place on cooling racks.

GENERAL QUESTIONS

1. How should brown sugar and solid fat be measured? Explain why these ingredients must be measured in this way.

2. What does it mean to "cream"?

3. Why should the oven rack be in the middle position when baking cookies?

4. Why were the cookies placed on cooling racks?

5. How important is exact oven temperature to baking quality?

LABORATORY 2

Food Preservation: Canning and Freezing

LABORATORY 2
FOOD PRESERVATION: CANNING AND FREEZING

The foods we eat should be wholesome, nutritious, and safe. This laboratory exercise will demonstrate to the student how to extend the shelf-life of food through canning and freezing.

VOCABULARY

antioxidant
blanch
boiling water bath process
freezer burn

high acid food
low acid food
polyphenoloxidase

pressure canner process
sterilization
turgor

OBJECTIVES

1. To demonstrate and observe the differences between raw pack and hot pack.
2. To demonstrate and discuss the differences between the boiling water bath process and the pressure canner process.
3. To define and demonstrate the differences between freezing fruits and vegetables as a simple method of preservation.
4. To prepare jellies, jams, conserves, and pickles as a form of preserving fruits and vegetables.

PRINCIPLES

1. The canning process to be used is determined by the pH of the food:
    a. High acid foods (pH <4.6) (fruits, pickles, jellies, jams, and some tomato varieties) are processed by the **boiling water bath** (212°F).
    b. Low acid foods (pH >4.6) (vegetables, poultry, meat, milk, fish, soups, etc.) are processed by the **pressure canner process** (240°F, at 10 pounds pressure).
2. **Time** and **temperature** are very important factors when canning. These two elements ensure that the product will be free of microorganisms and a sterile product is present. *FIG.1* illustrates the different temperatures and the survival rates of bacteria.
3. Foods processed under vacuum must be done so to insure destruction of *Clostridium botulinum*.
4. Food for canning can be packed either by raw pack or hot pack. Raw pack guarantees more food identity but more food will fit into the jar by the hot pack method.
5. Pickling of food involves vinegar (acid) and salt whereby the boiling water bath method will suffice in lowering the microbial load.
6. Jellies are made by a balanced formulation of fruit, pectin, acid, and sugar.
7. Enzymes are responsible for darkening sliced fruits and vegetables. Pretreatment of fruits and vegetables prior to freezing is necessary because freezing only slows down enzymatic activity.
8. Vegetables are blanched prior to freezing in order to inhibit enzyme action.
9. Fruits, because of their texture, cannot be blanched but are treated with an antioxidant prior to freezing.
10. Containers in which fruits or vegetables are stored for freezing must be tightly sealed in order to prevent freezer burn (sublimation).

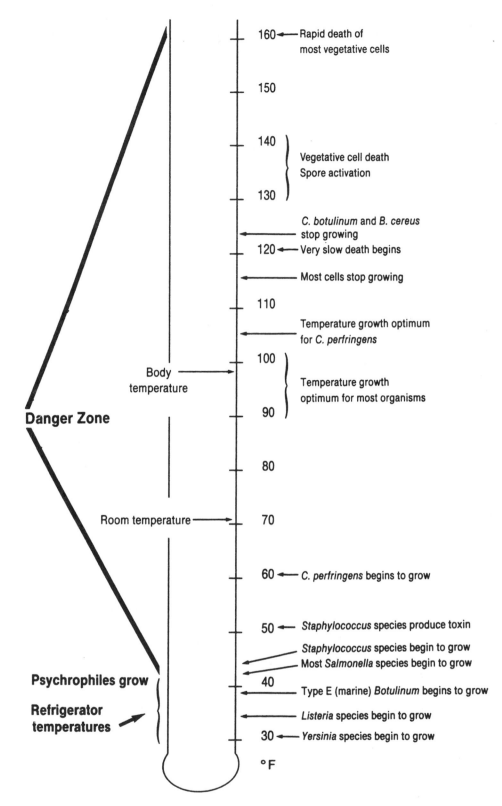

FIG.1. The growth of bacteria can be controlled by restricting the temperature at which foods are held. (Reprinted by permission from Eagan Press, *Food Safety*, 1992, p 110.)

I. OBSERVE AND LEARN HOW TO USE UTENSILS AND EQUIPMENT COMMONLY USED IN CANNING

A. JARS AND THEIR CLOSURES/TIN CANS

1. Check for and discard any glass jars with cracks or chips and any rings with dents or rust; these defects prevent air tight seals.
2. Wash jars in **hot soapy water** and **rinse well** (jars and rings are reusable).
3. Place lids in a pan of water; bring to a boil. Remove from heat and leave in hot water until ready to use. This softens the rubber on the lid and provides for an air tight seal.
   > Label each lid:
   > Food, Pack (if applicable), and Process
   > Date Canned
   > Laboratory Day and Time
   > Kitchen #

B. METHODS OF PACKING

1. Raw Pack: Uncooked food is packed into jars. The food is then covered with boiling liquid, leaving head space recommended (*FIG.2*).
2. Hot Pack: Food is heated in syrup, water, steam, or extracted juice. The hot food is then packed into jars and covered with boiling liquid, leaving head space recommended.

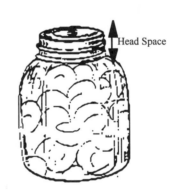

FIG.2. Head space prevents loss of liquid and effects seal in vacuum-type closures. (Reprinted with permission from Helen Charley, *Food Study Manual.* Ronald Press, NY.)

Head Space

C. PROCESSING EQUIPMENT

1. Water Bath: Select a deep container with a lid. Place a pint jar on a rack in the water bath canner. Water should be 1 to 2 inches above the top of the jar. Start timing when water boils. Boil gently for recommended time.
2. Pressure Canner: Put water in the canner to a depth of 2-3 inches. Place jars on rack in canner. Fasten lid securely. Open the pet cock and place the canner over the heat. Let the steam escape for 7-10 minutes in a steady stream. Close the pet cock and allow the pressure to build. Most foods are processed at 240°F at 10 pounds pressure. As soon as gauge registers this value, start timing and hold at 240°F for the allotted time. At the end of the processing time, turn off heat and allow gauge to return to zero (0) before opening canner and removing jars.

CAUTION: Always open the pet cock before attempting to remove the lid.

D. COOLING OF PROCESSED JARS

After jars are removed from the processing equipment, they are placed on a clean cloth. Allow some space between the jars for cooling and air circulation. Check the lids after cooling; the center of the lid should be depressed if sealed. If lids "pop" up and down when touched, they are to be reprocessed. After removing the ring, a sealed jar can be tipped without leakage.

QUESTIONS

1. What is the processing temperature in a water bath canner? Pressure canner?

2. What type of food is processed in a water bath canner? Why? A pressure canner? Why?

3. What is the purpose of 2-3 inches of water in the pressure canner?

4. Why should the pressure inside the canner be held steady?

II. FOODS TO BE PACKED AND PROCESSED

A. RAW PACKED TOMATOES (1 PINT JAR)

1. Prepare jar and lid as directed in Part I.
2. Wash 3 medium tomatoes. Loosen skins by dipping tomatoes into boiling water for about 30 seconds, then into cold water. Skins should slip off easily.
3. Cut tomatoes into quarters.
4. Place tomatoes into jar; add 1 teaspoon lemon juice and 1/4 teaspoon salt.
5. Pour boiling water into jar, leaving 1/2 inch headspace. Remove air bubbles by running spatula between jar and food.
6. Wipe jar rims. Cover with lids and screw on rings firmly, but not too tight. Label lid.
7. Process in boiling water bath for 45 minutes.

B. HOT PACKED TOMATOES (1 PINT JAR)

1. Prepare jar and lid as directed in Part I.
2. Wash 3 medium tomatoes. Loosen skins by dipping tomatoes into boilng water for about 30 seconds, then into cold water. Skins should slip off easily.
3. Cut tomatoes into quarters and place in saucepan. Add 1 teaspoon lemon juice. Bring to a boil; stir to prevent sticking.
4. Pack hot tomatoes into jar. Add 1/4 teaspoon salt (optional). Using juice from saucepan, fill jar with juice, leaving 1/2 inch head space. Remove air bubbles by running spatula between jar and food.
5. Wipe jar rims. Cover with lids and screw on rings firmly, but not too tight. Label lid.
6. Process in boiling water bath for 40 minutes.

C. APPLES (2 PINT JARS)

1. Prepare jars and lids as directed in Part I.
2. Wash, pare (peel), and slice 6 medium apples into 1/2 inch sections. Cut slices in half. In a large mixing bowl, dissolve 2 level tablespoons ascorbic acid powder ("Fruit Fresh") in 4 cups of water. Place apple chunks in this solution to prevent darkening.
3. Hot Pack in Water:
   a. Take half the apple chunks and put in a saucepan. Cover with water and bring to a boil. Add 1 tablespoon lemon juice. Boil for 5 minutes.

15

b. Pack apples into one pint jar. Quickly bring the water the apples were cooked in to a boil; fill jar with boiling apple water, leaving 1/2 inch head space. Remove air bubbles by running spatula between jar and food.

c. Wipe jar rim. Cover with lid and screw on ring firmly, but not too tight. Label lid.

d. Process in boiling water bath for 25 minutes.

4. Raw Pack in Water:

a. Pack apples into second pint jar. Quickly bring 2 cups water plus 1 tablespoon lemon juice to a boil; fill jar with hot water, leaving 1/2 inch head space. Remove air bubbles by running spatula between jar and food.

b. Wipe jar rim. Cover with lid and screw on ring firmly but not too tight. Label lid.

c. Process in boiling water bath for 30 minutes.

D. PEARS (2 PINT JARS)

1. Prepare jars and lids as directed in Part I.

2. Wash, pare (peel), cut in half, and core 6 medium pears. In a large mixing bowl, dissolve 2 level tablespoons ascorbic acid powder (Fruit Fresh) in 4 cups of water. Place pear halves in this solution to prevent darkening.

3. Make a syrup by heating 2 cups sugar and 4 cups water until sugar is dissolved.

4. Raw Pack in Syrup:

a. Pack half of pears into one pint jar. Add 1 tablespoon lemon juice. Bring syrup to a boil and fill jar with boiling syrup, leaving 1/2 inch head space. Remove air bubbles by running spatula between jar and food.

b. Wipe jar rim. Cover with lid and screw on ring firmly, but not too tight. Label lid.

c. Process in boiling water bath for 25 minutes.

5. Hot Pack in Syrup:

a. Add remaining pears to remaining syrup. Add 1 tablespoon lemon juice. Bring to a boil.

b. Pack hot pear halves into second pint jar. Quickly bring syrup to a boil; fill jar with boiling syrup, leaving 1/2 inch head space. Remove air bubbles by running spatula between jar and food.

c. Wipe jar rim. Cover with lid and screw on ring firmly, but not too tight. Label lid.

d. Process in boiling water for 20 minutes.

E. GREEN BEANS (2 PINT JARS)

1. Prepare jars and lids as directed in Part I.

2. Wash 3/4 pound green beans and drain. Cut or break off ends. Cut or break green beans into 1 to 1 1/2 inch pieces.

3. Raw Pack:

a. Pack raw beans tightly to 1/2 inch below top of one pint jar. Add 1/4 teaspoon salt (on top of beans).

b. Cover with boiling water, leaving 1/2 inch head space. Remove air bubbles by running spatula between jar and food.

c. Wipe jar rim. Cover with lid and screw on ring firmly, but not too tight. Label lid.

4. Hot Pack:

a. Cover cut beans with boiling water and cook for 5 minutes.

b. Pack hot beans loosely to 1/2 inch of top of second pint jar. Add 1/4 teaspoon salt.

c. Bring water beans were cooked in to a boil. Fill jar with boiling liquid, leaving 1/2 inch head space. Remove air bubbles by running spatula between jar and food.

d. Wipe jar rim. Cover with lid and screw on ring firmly, but not too tight. Label lid.

5. Process both jars in a pressure canner at 10 pounds pressure (240°F) for 30 minutes.

TABLE FOR EVALUATION OF CANNED PRODUCTS					
Food	Pack	Process	Jar Appearance	*Texture	*Flavor
Tomato	Raw				
Tomato	Hot				
Apples	Raw				
Apples	Hot				
Pears	Raw				
Pears	Hot				
Green Beans	Raw				
Green Beans	Hot				

*To be evaluated in a later lab.

F.   STRAWBERRY JAM (4 HALF-PINT JARS)

2 1/2 cups strawberries, crushed   2 tablespoons + 2 1/2 teaspoons powdered pectin ("Sure-Jel")
2 1/2 cups sugar

1.   Prepare jars and lids as directed in Part I.
2.   Crush strawberries. Put strawberries and powdered pectin in a large saucepan. Add 1 cup sugar.
3.   Bring berry mixture to a full boil over medium heat, stirring constantly. Immediately stir in the rest of the sugar.
4.   Stir and bring to a full rolling boil. Boil hard one minute, stirring constantly.
5.   Remove from heat. Skim off foam. Immediately ladle into jars, leaving 1/2 inch head space.
6.   Wipe jar rims. Cover with hot lids and screw on rings firmly, but not too tight. Label lid.
7.   Process in boiling water bath 10 minutes.

G.   FREEZER STRAWBERRY JAM (2 HALF-PINT JARS)

1 cup strawberries, crushed   2 tablespoons + 2 1/2 teaspoons powdered pectin ("Sure-Jel")
2 cups sugar   1/4 cup + 2 tablespoons water

1.   Prepare jars and lids as directed in Part I.
2.   Crush strawberries. Stir sugar into fruit and let stand 10 minutes.
3.   Mix powdered pectin and water in a small saucepan. Bring to a full boil and boil for one minute, stirring constantly.
4.   Immediately stir pectin mixture into fruit and continue to stir for 3 minutes.
5.   Ladle mixture into jars, leaving 1/2 inch head space. Wipe any spills from container. Cover with lid and screw on rings firmly, but not too tight. Label lid.
6.   Let stand at room temperature for 24 hours. Store jam in freezer.

H.   "LIGHT" GRAPE JELLY (3 HALF-PINT JARS)

2 cups grape juice   1 1/2 cups sugar
1/2 cup water   2 tablespoons + 2 1/2 teaspoons powdered "light" pectin

1.   Prepare jars and lids as directed in Part I.
2.   Thoroughly mix water and grape juice in a large saucepan.
3.   Measure sugar and set aside. Mix 2 tablespoons of measured sugar into powdered "light" pectin.

4. Stir the pectin-sugar mixture into juice in pan. Saucepan must be no more than 1/3 full to allow expansion space for full rolling boil.
5. Bring contents of saucepan to a full boil over medium heat, stirring constantly. Stir in remaining sugar.
6. Bring to a full rolling boil, stirring constantly and boil one minute.
7. Remove from heat. Skim off foam. Pour into hot jars, leaving 1/2 inch head space.
8. Wipe jar rims. Cover with hot lids and screw rings on firmly, but not too tight. Label lid.
9. Process in boiling water bath 10 minutes.

TABLE FOR EVALUATION OF JELLY/JAM			
Product	Clarity	Flavor*	Texture*
Strawberry Jam			
Freezer Strawberry Jam			
"Light" Grape Jelly			

*To be evaluated in a later lab.

QUESTIONS

1. What is head space? Why is it important?

2. Compare the processing times for raw pack and hot pack food items and account for the differences.

3. What are the main ingredients for making jelly? What causes the pectin to set?

4. Under what conditions are *Clostridium botulinum* spores destroyed?

5. What may cause liquid to be lost from jars during canning? Can you open the jar and pour some liquid back after processing?

III. FREEZING OF FRUITS AND VEGETABLES

A. TO SHOW THE EFFECTS OF BLANCHING ON THE QUALITY OF FROZEN VEGETABLES

1. Prepare for freezing 1/4 pound of the following: carrot, broccoli, or cauliflower. Pick over vegetables carefully; discard any rotten or decayed parts; wash and dry thoroughly.
2. Blanch 1/2 of the assigned vegetable:
   a. Place vegetable in basket or strainer.
   b. Plunge basket into boiling water. Water must be boiling and vegetable must be totally covered.
   c. Blanch carrot for 3 minutes; blanch broccoli (flowerets) for 3 minutes; blanch cauliflower (1 inch pieces) for 3 minutes. Then plunge the blanched vegetable in ice water.
3. Leave the other half of the assigned vegetable unblanched.

4. Pack unblanched and blanched vegetable, separately, in small plastic bags; seal and label.
5. Freeze at 0°F (-18°C) and hold in frozen storage, preferably 3 weeks or longer.
6.* Cook the two lots of frozen vegetables until tender in a small amount of boiling, salted water.
7. Evaluate the two lots of vegetables for the characteristics listed in the table provided.

*After storage for 3 weeks or more.

TABLE FOR EVALUATION OF UNBLANCHED/BLANCHED VEGETABLES					
Vegetable	Treatment	Color	Aroma	Taste	Texture
Carrot	Unblanched				
	Blanched				
Broccoli	Unblanched				
	Blanched				
Cauliflower	Unblanched				
	Blanched				

QUESTIONS

1. Why should vegetables be blanched before they are frozen?

2. Why were the vegetables plunged in ice water after blanching?

B. TO SHOW THE EFFECTS OF VARIOUS TREATMENTS ON THE QUALITY OF FROZEN FRUIT

1. Wash, pare, and slice 6 apples and divide into 6 equal portions (one apple for each treatment). Treat as indicated below:
2. Dry Pack
   a. Leave 1 cut apple untreated.
   b. Blanch the second apple for 2 minutes. Cool in cold water. Drain.
   c. Mix 2 tablespoons sugar with the third cut up apple.
   d. Mix 2 tablespoons sugar and 1/8 teaspoon citric acid with the fourth cut up apple.
3. Syrup Pack (40% Sugar Syrup: 3 cups sugar and 4 cups water. Mix sugar and water together until sugar dissolves.)
   a. To one-half cup of the 40% syrup, add 1/16 teaspoon of citric acid and cover the fifth apple.
   b. For the sixth apple cover with 1/2 cup of 40% syrup.
4. Packaging and Freezing
   a. Pack into freezer bags; seal and label.
   b. Freeze at 0°F and hold in frozen storage, preferably 3 weeks or longer.
   c. Remove from the freezer and thaw, sealed, in the refrigerator (4-6 hours) or under cold running water for approximately 1 hour.
   d. Rank the 6 samples for color, texture, and flavor in the table provided.

TABLE FOR EVALUATION OF FROZEN APPLES			
Treatment	Color	Texture	Flavor
Dry Pack			
Plain			
Blanched			
Sugar			
Sugar and citric acid			
Syrup Pack			
40% syrup			
40% syrup with citric acid			

QUESTIONS

1. What causes browning of apples?

2. How can browning be prevented?

3. Which treatment will have the best effect?

4. How will blanching affect the fruit?

5. Why were the bags tightly sealed before the vegetable or fruit was frozen?

6. How may fluctuations of storage temperature affect the quality of frozen foods?

LABORATORY 3

Starch and Cereal Cookery:

Role of Gelatinization and Gelation

LABORATORY 3
STARCH AND CEREAL COOKERY:
ROLE OF GELATINIZATION AND GELATION

Starch is a term used to indicate both individual molecules and the collection of these molecules organized as granules. Starch grains are used as thickening agents in soups and sauces. Cereal cookery is basically starch cookery, as starch makes up the major portion of the cereal grain. The first part of this laboratory exercise is to provide some basis for an understanding of the behavior of starch when used as a thickening agent. The second part stresses the cooking of various cereal grains which were processed under different conditions.

VOCABULARY

al dente	dextrin	germ	roux
amylopectin	endosperm	grits	semolina
amylose	enriched	instant cereal	suspension
bran	gelatinization	oatmeal	viscosity
cornmeal	gelation	quick cooking	waxy starch
converted			

OBJECTIVES

1. To study the effects of heat on the cooking properties of starch.
2. To differentiate between gelatinization and gelation.
3. To examine the effects of time, temperature, agitation, acidity, and ingredients on the gelatinization and gelation properties of starch.
4. To recognize and understand that cereal cookery is basically the gelatinization of starch.

PRINCIPLES

1. When starch and water are mixed together a temporary suspension is formed.
2. When moist heat is applied the starch granules swell up to a certain point and a colloidal dispersion is formed. This is called gelatinization.
3. There is an increase in viscosity and this is attributed to amylopectin.
4. The gelling of the dispersion is attributed to the amylose.
5. Heat, time, agitation, acid, and other ingredients will have an effect on gelatinization and gelation.
6. Cereal grains are cooked in water until they become hydrated, tender, and soft in the process of gelatinization.
7. Cooking grains in only the amount of water that will be absorbed when they are fully hydrated permits maximum retention of nutrients and prevents deleterious color changes.
8. The cooking time for cereal products (grains, rice, pasta) depends on the size and characteristics of the grain or pasta.

I. STARCH PRINCIPLES

A. TO SHOW FACTORS WHICH AFFECT THE THICKNESS OF A COOKED STARCH PASTE

As influenced by the kind of starch.
As influenced by sugar, acid, and dextrinization.

1. Use pans of the same size.
2. Use 1 cup water for each starch listed except #5 in the following table, and for this use 2/3 cup water and 1/3 cup + 2 tablespoons freshly squeezed lemon juice.

3. Mix the starch with a small amount of the liquid to form a smooth paste. Add the remainder of the water and bring to a boil; cook directly over medium heat, stirring continuously.
4. Remove from heat.
5. Pour approximately 3/4 cup of cooked starch paste into a custard cup.
6. Let stand to cool.
7. Unmold onto small plate and record observations in the table provided.

TABLE FOR EVALUATION OF STARCH GELS				
			Cooled Paste	
No.	Kind of Starch	Amount of Starch (Tablespoon)	Firmness	Appearance
1	Flour	2		
2	Cornstarch	1		
3	Cornstarch	2		
4	Modified food starch	2		
5	Cornstarch, water, and lemon juice	2		
6	Flour, lightly browned	2		
7	Flour, darkly browned	2		
8	Cornstarch and 1/3 cup sugar	2		

QUESTIONS

1. Is there a difference in the thickening effect between flour and cornstarch?

2. How would you recommend the addition of an acid to a starch paste?

3. What effect did the dry heat have on the flour? Did time and temperature have an effect on gelatinization and viscosity?

4. What effect does sugar have on the gelatinization of starch?

5. Differentiate between gelatinization and gelation.

B. TO STUDY THE EFFECT OF WATER TEMPERATURE ON STARCH DISPERSION

1. Cold water:
   a. Stir 1 tablespoon of flour into 8 oz. of cold water in your glass measuring cup. Record your observations.

   _____
   _____

   b. Allow glass to stand for 10 minutes. Record your observations.

   _____
   _____

2. Boiling water:
   a. Bring 1 cup of water to a boil in a 1 quart saucepan. Add 1 tablespoon flour to the boiling water. Stir vigorously. Record your observations.

   _____
   _____

QUESTIONS

1. What causes the lumps in the solution?

2. Why does the flour settle to the bottom of the container?

C. TO SHOW THE EFFECTS OF THE PROPORTIONS OF FLOUR TO MILK ON THE CONSISTENCY OF WHITE SAUCE

1. Prepare each of the white sauces, using **fluid skim milk**.
2. Compare the white sauces for thicknesses.

BASIC WHITE SAUCE PROPORTIONS					
Kind	Flour	Fat	Salt	Liquid	Uses
Thin	1 tablespoon	1 tablespoon	1/4 teaspoon	1 cup	Cream soups made from starch foods
Medium	2 tablespoons	2 tablespoons	1/4 teaspoon	1 cup	Creamed dishes, scalloped dishes, gravy
Thick	3 tablespoons	2 tablespoons	1/2 teaspoon	1 cup	Cooked salad dressing; souffles
Very thick	4 tablespoons	2 1/2 tablespoons	1/2 teaspoon	1 cup	Croquettes

D. METHOD 1

1. Melt fat over low heat. Add flour and seasonings and blend.
2. Remove pan from heat; gradually add liquid.
3. Cook over medium heat, stirring continuously until mixture thickens.
4. Bring mixture to a boil and boil for 1 minute.

E. METHOD 2 (LOW-FAT METHOD)

1. Blend the flour and salt with 1/4 cup cold milk. Stir until all lumps have been separated.
2. Add remaining milk. Stir thoroughly.
3. Place the mixture in a saucepan over direct heat; stir constantly over low heat until mixture boils; boil for 1 minute.
4. As the mixture boils, add 1/2 of the fat indicated for type of sauce being prepared. Stir thoroughly until fat is blended into the sauce.

TABLE FOR EVALUATION OF WHITE SAUCE			
Type	Method	Appearance	Texture/Consistency
Thin	1		
	2		
Medium	1		
	2		
Thick	1		
	2		
Very Thick	1		
	2		

CHARACTERISTICS OF HIGH QUALITY WHITE SAUCES

Appearance:	*White to creamy (dependent on type of fat used); opaque.*
Consistency:	*Smooth; even starch gelatinization and distribution.*
Thin:	*Flows freely; like thin cream.*
Medium:	*Fluid, but thick; flows slowly; like heavy cream.*
Thick:	*Thick; holds imprint of spoon.*
Very Thick:	*Will not flow; holds cut edge.*
Flavor:	*Very bland; fat used may vary flavor.*

QUESTIONS

1.   What is the roux method?

2.   Why is the sauce boiled for 1 minute?

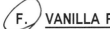

VANILLA PUDDING (CONVENTIONAL METHOD)

1 tablespoon cornstarch	2 egg yolks
2 tablespoons sugar	1/8 teaspoon salt
1 cup milk	1/2 teaspoon vanilla

1.   Mix together cornstarch and sugar.
2.   Add milk, egg yolks, and salt; stir to blend (use whisk to blend well).
3.   Cook over medium heat, stirring constantly.
4.   Bring mixture to a boil and boil 1 minute.
5.   Remove from heat and stir in vanilla.
6.   Pour into custard cup and cool.
7.   Compare to other puddings.

MICROWAVE PUDDING

1.   Use ingredients for conventional Vanilla Pudding.
2.   Mix dry ingredients in a quart measuring cup.
3.   Gradually stir in milk and egg yolks; continue stirring until thoroughly mixed.
4.   Microwave uncovered on high for 3 minutes.

5. Stir well. Microwave on high for 3 minutes more.
6. Remove; stir in vanilla.
7. Pour into serving dish.
8. Compare to other puddings.

H. INSTANT PUDDING MIX

1. Prepare a vanilla pudding mix according to package directions and compare to the pudding above.

I. COMMERCIALLY CANNED PUDDING

1. Compare a commercially canned pudding to the other puddings.

TABLE FOR EVALUATION OF PUDDING			
Pudding	Appearance	Taste	Consistency
Conventional			
Microwaved			
Instant Mix			
Commercially Canned			

CHARACTERISTICS OF HIGH QUALITY PUDDING

Appearance: Moist and shiny; film will form on top as pudding cools.
Consistency: Pudding should be firm but not hard.
Flavor: Slightly sweet.

QUESTIONS

1. What is the difference between the puddings?

    flavor?

    texture?

    ease of preparation?

2. How can you prevent the skin from forming on the surface of the puddings?

3. What causes the pudding to set as it cools?

4. What would happen if the pudding was stored in the refrigerator for a long period of a time?

II. CEREAL COOKERY

A. TO DEMONSTRATE AND COMPARE THE BEHAVIOR OF STARCH IN CEREAL PRODUCTS

1. **Cereals**
   a. *Bulgur wheat (sometimes called parboiled wheat):* Whole wheat that has been cooked, dried, partly debranned, and cracked into coarse, angular fragments. Originated in the Near East.
      1. Prepare following directions on package.
   b. *Farina (granulated wheat endosperm):* Made from wheat other than durum with the bran and most of the germ removed. It is prepared by grinding and sifting the wheat to a granular form (marketed as Cream of Wheat).
      1. Prepare following directions on package.
   c. *Oatmeal (rolled oats):* Made by rolling the grouts (oats with hull removed) to form flakes. Quick-cooking oats are cut into tiny particles which are then rolled into thin, small flakes. Instant oatmeal has been precooked.
      1. Prepare following directions on package.
   d. *Hominy grits (corn grits, grits):* Prepared from either white or yellow corn from which the bran and the germ have been removed. The remaining edible portion is ground and sifted. Grits are coarser than cornmeal.
      1. Prepare following directions on package.
   e. *Cornmeal:* Prepared by grinding cleaned white or yellow corn to a fineness specified by federal standards. Cornmeal may be bolted (further decreases size of granule); it may be degerminated (remove germ portion of kernel thus removing fat); it may be enriched (add specified amounts of thiamin, riboflavin, niacin, and iron; optional: calcium, vitamin D).
      1. Prepare recipe for cornmeal mush (Recipe B).

B. CORNMEAL MUSH

1/2 cup cornmeal	1 1/2 cups boiling water
1/2 cup cold water	1/2 teaspoon salt

1. Bring 1 1/2 cups water to a boil.
2. Blend the cornmeal, salt, and 1/2 cup cold water together.
3. Remove boiling water from heat; spoon or pour the cornmeal mixture into hot water; stir until blended.
4. Return to heat and bring to a boil; boil for 5 minutes.
5. Reduce heat to lowest temperature. Cover; allow to heat for 10 minutes more.

CHARACTERISTICS OF HIGH QUALITY COOKED CEREALS

Appearance:	Distinct particles, granules, or flakes.
Consistency:	Thick; somewhat viscous (without gumminess).
Flavor:	Bland (cooked starch); typical for grain (wheat, corn, oats); well rounded (no raw starch).
Mouth Feel:	Particles remain discrete; soft.

TABLE FOR EVALUATION OF CEREALS			
Cereal	Appearance	Consistency	Taste
Oat Bran			
Farina, Instant			
Farina, Regular			
Oatmeal, Instant			
Oatmeal, Regular			
Oatmeal, Quick Cooking			
Grits, Instant			
Grits, Regular			
Cornmeal, White			
Cornmeal, Yellow			

C. BULGUR PILAF

1 cup bulgur wheat
1 medium onion, chopped
1/2 cup celery, chopped

3 tablespoons margarine
2 cups chicken broth
1/4 teaspoon salt

1. In a skillet, saute bulgur wheat , onion, and celery in margarine.
2. Add broth and salt.
3. Cover and bring to a boil, reduce heat, and simmer for 15 minutes.

D. RICE

1. Steamed Rice

1/2 cup rice*   1/4 teaspoon salt
1 cup water

*For converted rice follow recipe on package.

1. Add salt to water and bring to a rolling boil.
2. Stir in the rice.
3. Heat until the water returns to boiling. Then lower heat to simmering; cover pan tightly and cook rice very slowly for 15 minutes. Remove from heat and allow to stand for 5 minutes.
4. Measure the cooked rice to obtain increase in volume: 1/2 cup raw rice yields _____ cups cooked rice.

TABLE FOR EVALUATION OF RICE			
Rice	Appearance	Texture	Flavor
Long Grain			
Medium Grain			
Short Grain			

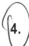

2. Rice Pilaf

2 tablespoons butter or margarine
1 small onion, finely chopped
1 cup long-grain converted rice

2 cups water
2 beef or chicken bouillon cubes
dash of pepper

1. Melt margarine in a heavy 2 quart saucepan.
2. Saute onion over low heat until soft and translucent.
3. Add rice and cook for a few minutes until a light brown.
4. Add pepper, water, and bouillon. Bring water to a boil; then lower to a simmer and cover with a tight fitting cover.
5. Cook for 15-20 minutes. Remove from heat and allow rice to stand for 5 minutes. Fluff with a fork.

3. Curried Rice Pilaf

2 tablespoons vegetable oil
1 large onion, thinly sliced
1 1/2 teaspoons curry powder
1 1/2 cups basmati OR Texmati OR long grain
    white rice

1 cinnamon stick
3 cups chicken broth
1 medium red pepper, cored, seeded, thinly sliced
1 small carrot, pared and shredded
1/2 cup whole kernel corn, defrosted

1. Heat oil in large skillet over medium heat. Add onion; saute until browned, about 7 minutes.
2. Stir in curry powder and rice.
3. Add cinnamon stick and broth.
4. Bring to boiling. Lower heat; cover and simmer 10 minutes.
5. Add shredded carrot, red pepper, and kernel corn; cover for 5 minutes, simmering.
6. Remove from heat and let stand, covered, 10 minutes.

4. Fried Rice

1/4 cup chopped onion
2 tablespoons chopped green pepper
2 tablespoons salad oil
2 cups cooked rice*

1 can (5 ounces) water chestnuts, drained and sliced
4 ounces sliced fresh mushrooms
2 tablespoons soy sauce
3 eggs, beaten

1. In a large skillet, cook and stir onion, mushrooms, and green pepper in oil until onion is tender.
2. Stir in rice, water chestnuts, and soy sauce.
3. Cook over low heat 10 minutes, stirring frequently.
4. Stir in beaten eggs; cook and stir 2-3 minutes longer.
*Rice must have been cooked and cooled thoroughly before using in recipe.

CHARACTERISTICS OF HIGH QUALITY COOKED RICE

Appearance:	*Grains intact; white, translucent.*
Texture:	*Grains firm, but tender; fluffy.*
Flavor:	*Bland.*

QUESTIONS

1. Why does the amount of water used to cook cereals vary?

2. Describe the characteristics of the bran, germ, and endosperm of the cereal grain.

3. Describe how and why starting rice to cook in cold water and in boiling water affect the texture of the cooked rice.

E. **PASTA**

1. **Neopolitan Casserole**

3/4 pound ground turkey
1/2 cup onion, finely chopped
1/2 cup green pepper, chopped
1 garlic clove, crushed
1/2 teaspoon dried basil
1/2 teaspoon oregano
1/2 teaspoon fennel seed
1/8 teaspoon crushed red pepper flakes

1 tablespoon sugar
3/4 teaspoon salt
1 can (1 pound 14 ounce) Italian style tomatoes, undrained
1/2 pound fresh spinach or 1 (10 ounce) package frozen
    chopped spinach (defrosted and drained well)
1/4 pound medium shell macaroni
1/2 cup low-fat mozzarella cheese, grated

1. Saute ground turkey, onion, green pepper, garlic, basil, oregano, fennel seed, and red pepper flakes; stir frequently until meat is browned and vegetables are tender - about 20 minutes. Drain off fat.
2. Add sugar, salt, and tomatoes. Mash tomatoes with a wooden spoon. Bring to boiling. Reduce heat; simmer uncovered and stir occasionally until thickened - about 20 minutes.
3. Wash spinach thoroughly and remove stems. Place in a large kettle with some water. Cook, covered, and stir occasionally, 4-6 minutes or until leaves are wilted. **Drain well**; reserve.
4. Preheat oven to 350°F.
5. In a large kettle, cook shell macaroni until al dente; drain well. In large kettle or bowl combine sauce, spinach, and shell macaroni; toss lightly to mix well. Turn out into a 1 1/2 quart casserole.
6. Sprinkle with grated mozzarella cheese. Bake uncovered 30 minutes or until bubbly and lightly browned.

2. **Baked Ziti with Vegetables**

2 tablespoons olive oil
1 medium-sized sweet green pepper, cored,
    seeded, and diced
1 medium-sized red pepper, cored, seeded, and
    diced
1 medium-sized yellow pepper, cored, seeded, and
    diced
2 large cloves garlic, freshly chopped
2 large onions, coarsely chopped
1/4 pound mushrooms, chopped

1 can (16 ounces) whole tomatoes, undrained
1 can (8 ounces) tomato sauce
1 teaspoon leaf basil, crumbled
1/2 teaspoon salt
1/4 teaspoon pepper
1/4 teaspoon leaf oregano
1/2 pound fresh spinach, cleaned and stemmed
8 ounces ziti, cooked according to package directions
1 container (8 ounces) part-skim ricotta cheese
1/4 cup grated Parmesan cheese

1. Heat 1 tablespoon oil in large skillet over medium heat. Add green, red, and yellow pepper; saute until barely tender, about 5 minutes. Remove with slotted spoon and set aside.
2. Heat remaining tablespoon oil in skillet. Add onion; saute until softened, 4-5 minutes. Add garlic and mushrooms; saute 2 minutes.
3. Break up tomatoes with fork and add with liquid to skillet along with tomato sauce, basil, salt, pepper, and oregano. Bring to boiling. Lower heat; simmer uncovered until slightly thickened, about 20 minutes. Add spinach; cook, stirring, until the spinach wilts.
4. Preheat oven to 350°F. Spray 2 1/2 quart casserole with non-stick vegetable spray.

5. Combine ziti, tomato mixture, ricotta, and 2/3 of peppers in a large bowl. Spoon mixture into prepared casserole. Sprinkle with Parmesan cheese. Bake for 25 minutes. Sprinkle with remaining peppers.

3. Marinara Sauce

2 tablespoons olive oil
2-3 garlic cloves, finely chopped
1/3 cup parsley, chopped
1/2 teaspoon salt
1 can (28 ounces) Italian tomatoes

1/2 teaspoon oregano
1/2 teaspoon basil
dash pepper
8 ounces (1/2 pound) spaghetti, cooked

1. Saute oil, garlic, and parsley for 3 minutes.
2. Add tomatoes, oregano, basil, salt, and pepper. Mash tomatoes with a fork.
3. Simmer uncovered for about 30 minutes or until thickened.
4. Serve over hot cooked spaghetti.

4. Noodles Alfredo

2 tablespoons margarine
1 tablespoon flour
1/4 teaspoon salt
1 1/2 cups skim milk
dash of black pepper

dash of grated nutmeg
1/2 cup Parmesan cheese, grated
2 tablespoons butter or margarine
8 ounces (1/2 pound) fettucine noodles, cooked and drained

1. In a 2 quart saucepan, melt margarine. Add flour and salt. Remove from heat.
2. Slowly add skim milk; stir until ingredients are combined. Return to heat; add black pepper and nutmeg.
3. Bring mixture to a boil over low heat; stirring constantly. Boil for 1 minute.
4. In the meantime, cook fettucine noodles in a large kettle according to package directions; drain well.
5. In a large bowl combine sauce, noodles, 2 tablespoons margarine, and Parmesan cheese. Toss lightly making sure noodles are coated with sauce. Lightly sprinkle with extra black pepper or Parmesan cheese, if desired, and serve.

CHARACTERISTICS OF HIGH QUALITY PASTA

Appearance: Distinct strands or pieces.
Tenderness: Tender; little resistance to bite.
Flavor: Bland; noodles may have a slight egg flavor.

GENERAL QUESTIONS

1. Why is cooked long grain rice fluffier than short grain rice?

   Under what circumstances would each of these be used?

2. What is the difference between:

   a. grits and cornmeal?

b.   regular, instant, and quick-cooking oatmeal?

c.   long grain rice and converted rice?

3.   Why must pasta be cooked in a large amount of water?

4.   What is the difference in ingredients between various pasta products?

5.   What is enrichment and why are cereal products enriched?

6.   To what degree should pasta be cooked when it is to be used in a casserole recipe?

LABORATORY 4

Quick and Yeast Breads:

Role of Manipulation and Gluten Formation in Doughs

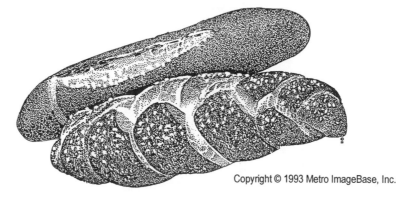

LABORATORY 4
QUICK AND YEAST BREADS: ROLE OF MANIPULATION AND GLUTEN FORMATION IN DOUGHS

Bread has an integral role in the diet. There are quick breads (biscuits, muffins, etc.) which require very little manipulation, thereby having little gluten formation, and are leavened by baking powder and/or baking soda. Yeast bread requires a longer mixing time, greater gluten formation, and requires yeast as the leavening agent. This laboratory exercise will introduce the student to the making of these various breads. The exercise will emphasize the various leavening agents used, as well as, the selection of various flours and their roles in the structural formation in the breads.

VOCABULARY

all-purpose flour	bread flour	gluten	oven-spring
baking powder	cut in	glutenin	proofing
baking soda	fermentation	knead	soft wheat flour
biscuit method	gliadin	muffin method	yeast

OBJECTIVES

1. To study the effect of manipulation on gluten development in quick breads.
2. To identify the gluten forming properties of various wheat flours.
3. To learn how different leavening agents affect volume and structural development in both quick and yeast breads.

PRINCIPLES

1. Gluten, which gives structure to any baked product, is made up of gliadin and glutenin.
2. The strength of the gluten formation is dependent on
   a. the amount of protein in the wheat flour.
   b. the amount of manipulation.
3. Muffins and biscuits require very little mixing for gluten development.
4. Muffin ingredients (liquid added to dry ingredients) are stirred for about 15 strokes.
5. Biscuit dough is kneaded for 10 strokes and the dough is rolled 1/2-3/4 inch thickness for cutting biscuits.
6. Yeast bread dough is kneaded for 8 minutes to
   a. develop gluten.
   b. distribute the ingredients.
7. One important ingredient in bread dough is yeast.
8. Yeast is allowed to ferment and this causes the dough to rise.
9. The temperature of the water should be between 105-115°F to ensure complete activity of the yeast.

I. **TO EVALUATE FACTORS WHICH AFFECT THE QUALITY OF MUFFINS**

A. **MUFFINS (BASIC RECIPE)**

2 cups all-purpose flour
1 teaspoon salt
3 teaspoons double-acting baking powder
2 tablespoons sugar

2 tablespoons oil
1 egg
1 cup milk

1. Sift together flour, salt, baking powder, and sugar into a bowl.
2. Blend together thoroughly egg, oil, and milk and pour into dry ingredients.

34

3. Combine with only enough stirring to barely dampen dry ingredients. Batter will be lumpy.
4. Fill greased muffin cups 2/3 full.
5. Bake at 400°F for 20-25 minutes. Yield: 12 medium muffins.
6 Variations in Manipulation (*FIG.1*)
    a.   In step 3, stir batter **7 strokes** and then spoon two (2) muffins into the tin.
    b.   Stir **4 more strokes** and spoon two (2) more muffins into the tins.
    c.   Stir an **additional 4 strokes** and spoon two (2) more muffins into the tins.
    d.   Stir **5 more strokes** or until smooth and shiny. Spoon into last two muffin tins.
7. Variation using maximum amount of fat and sugar
    a.   Use mixing variations as above.
    b.   Substitute in basic recipe:
        1.   Use 4 tablespoons sugar and 4 tablespoons oil.
8. Record all observations in table provided.

(A)   (B)   (C)

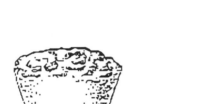 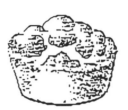 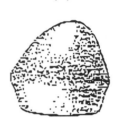

FIG.1. Undermixed (A); optimum (B); and overmixed (C) muffins. (Reprinted with permission from Helen Charley, *Food Study Manual*, Ronald Press, NY.)

TABLE FOR EVALUATION OF MUFFINS				
Variation	7 Strokes	11 Strokes	15 Strokes	20 Strokes
Regular Recipe				
Extra Fat and Sugar				

CHARACTERISTICS OF HIGH QUALITY MUFFINS	
Color:	*Golden brown exterior.*
External Appearance:	*Slightly rounded, pebbly tops.*
Texture:	*Tender and light.*
Structure:	*Even-textured with medium, round holes; slightly moist.*

QUESTIONS

1. Describe the method in making muffins.

2. How are muffins leavened?

3. Define and give chemical reaction for double-acting baking powder.

4. How does under and over manipulation affect leavening action?

5. Describe how added amounts of fat and sugar affect the muffin. Why?

II. TO EVALUATE FACTORS WHICH AFFECT THE QUALITY OF BISCUITS

A. BASIC BISCUIT RECIPE

2 cups all-purpose flour   5 tablespoons fat
3/4 teaspoon salt   2/3-3/4 cup milk (approximately)
3 teaspoons double-acting baking powder

1. Sift flour, salt, and baking powder together in a bowl.
2. Cut in fat (using pastry blender or two knives) until mixture looks like coarse corn meal.
3. Add milk to make a soft dough and stir rapidly with a fork until the mixture thickens.
4. Turn onto a lightly floured board and knead 10 times.
5. Roll out to 1/2-3/4 inch thickness.
6. Cut with a floured cutter (2-2 1/2 inches in diameter). Cut straight down into dough and lift straight out. Use even pressure in cutting down on the dough to get more evenly shaped biscuits. Do not twist.
7. Bake at 425°F for 10-12 minutes or until lightly browned.

B. BUTTERMILK BISCUITS

1 1/2 cups all-purpose flour   1/2 teaspoon salt
1 teaspoon baking powder   1/4 cup shortening
1/2 teaspoon baking soda   2/3 cup buttermilk (approximately)

1. Sift together flour, baking powder, baking soda, and salt.
2. Cut in shortening with a pastry blender until it resembles coarse corn meal.
3. Add milk to form a soft dough and stir rapidly with a fork until the mixture thickens.
4. Turn onto a lightly floured board and knead 10 times.
5. Roll out to 1/2-3/4 inch thickness.
6. Cut with a floured cutter. Use even pressure when cutting down on the dough to get evenly shaped biscuits. Do not twist.
7. Bake on an ungreased sheet at 425°F for 10-12 minutes.

C. LOW-FAT BUTTERMILK BISCUITS
(Reprinted by permission of Southern Progress Corporation, *Cooking Light* Magazine, September 1993, p. 110-111.)

2 cups all-purpose flour   1/4 teaspoon salt
2 teaspoons baking powder   3 tablespoons plus 1 teaspoon chilled stick margarine, cut into small pieces
1/4 teaspoon baking soda   3/4 cup 1% low-fat buttermilk

1. Combine flour and next three ingredients in a bowl; cut in chilled margarine with a pastry blender until the mixture resembles coarse meal.
2. Add buttermilk and stir just until dry ingredients are moistened.
3. Turn dough out onto a floured surface; knead 4-5 times.
4. Roll dough to a 1/2 inch thickness; cut with a 2 1/2 inch biscuit cutter.
5. Bake at 450° for 12 minutes or until golden.

D. WHIPPING CREAM BISCUITS

2 cups self-rising soft wheat flour   1 cup whipping cream

1. Combine ingredients, stirring with a fork until blended (dough will be stiff).
2. Turn dough out onto a lightly floured surface and knead 10-12 times.
3. Roll out to 1/2 inch thickness; cut with a floured biscuit cutter. Use even pressure in cutting down on the dough to get more evenly shaped biscuits. Do not twist.
4. Bake at 450°F on a lightly greased baking sheet for 10-12 minutes.

TABLE FOR EVALUATION OF BISCUITS			
Biscuit	Flakiness	Tenderness	Flavor
Basic			
Buttermilk			
Low-Fat			
Whipping Cream			

CHARACTERISTICS OF HIGH QUALITY BISCUITS

Color: Light and golden.
Volume: High and fairly smooth, level tops (Fig.2).
Texture: Tender and light.
Structure: Flaky and slightly moist.

(A)   (B)   (C)

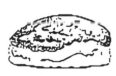 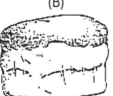 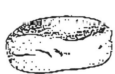

FIG.2. Undermanipulated (A), optimum (B), and overmanipulated (C) biscuits. (Reprinted with permission from Helen Charley, *Food Study Manual*, Ronald Press, NY.)

QUESTIONS

1. What is the method used for mixing biscuits?

   How does it differ from the method for making muffins?

2. What would happen if a biscuit was overkneaded?

3. Describe the role of baking soda in biscuits made with buttermilk.

III. TO IDENTIFY THE GLUTEN FORMING PROPERTIES OF VARIOUS WHEAT FLOURS

 A. **GLUTEN BALLS**

(Note: Instructor should list types of flours which will illustrate various degrees of gluten development; such as, all-purpose flour, bread flour, cake flour, whole wheat flour, etc.)

1. Measure 1 cup flour of each type. Add just enough water (about 1/4 cup) to form a stiff dough. Rub the wetted flour around the sides of the bowl to incorporate any fragments into the dough. Knead the ball of dough for about 15 minutes to develop the gluten.
2. Fill the bowl with cool water and knead the dough under water to wash out the starch components. Change the water as needed, using care to retain all the gluten. (Or, carefully wash under running water. Place a strainer under gluten ball to collect any pieces. Add back to the ball.)
3. **Washing** is **completed** when the **water squeezed** from the mass is **clear**.
4. Bake at 400°F for 15 minutes; reduce the heat to 300°F and continue baking for 40 minutes. Record observations in table provided.

TABLE FOR EVALUATION OF GLUTEN BALLS	
Type of Flour	Observations

QUESTIONS

1. What is the relationship of the size of the gluten ball to the type of flour and amount of protein?

2. What does the gluten ball reveal as to the flour's baking ability?

IV. TO STUDY FACTORS WHICH AFFECT THE QUALITY OF YEAST BREAD

 A. **BASIC YEAST DOUGH**

1/2 cup warm water (105°F-115°F, or 40°C) 2 cups all-purpose flour*
1 tablespoon sugar   1/2 teaspoon salt
2 tablespoons dried milk solids   2 tablespoons shortening
1 package quick rising yeast   1 egg

1. Preheat oven to 400°F.
2. Measure the sugar and dried milk solids.
3. Measure the water and place in a 2 quart bowl. Add the yeast. Stir until blended. Add the sugar and the dried milk solids. Stir until blended. Allow this yeast mixture to stand while measuring the remaining ingredients (5-10 minutes). The yeast activity is initiated.

4. Measure remaining ingredients.
5. Add the egg and 1 cup of the flour to the yeast mixture. Beat until the batter is smooth (about 100 strokes).
6. Add the salt, shortening, and half of the remaining flour; stir until well blended.
7. If the dough is still too sticky to turn out on a lightly floured board, add the remaining portion of flour and stir into dough. If the dough is not sticky use the flour that was not put into the dough to lightly flour the breadboard.
8. Put the dough onto the lightly floured board. Knead the dough until it is lightly blistered under the dough (about 8-10 minutes of kneading); the dough has a satiny sheen; the dough has become resilient - when pinched lightly with the finger, the dough springs back.
9. Place the dough in a lightly greased bowl; lightly grease the surface of the dough. Allow dough to rise at least 20 minutes - to double in bulk is preferable when time permits. Cover the bowl with plastic wrap and then place bowl over another bowl filled partly with warm water. Dough is fermented fully when 2 fingers leave an indentation in the dough.
10. Lightly knead the dough for 1 minute to evenly distribute the gas cells.
11. Weigh out 75 grams of dough. Shape into a bread loaf and place in a small greased bread pan (4 1/2 × 2 1/2 inches). Shape the remaining dough into crescent rolls, clover leaf rolls, or any other shapes you desire (*FIG.3*).
12. Allow the loaf of bread and shaped rolls to rise until double in bulk. This may take 20 minutes or longer; do not have rolls in too warm a place for this second rising. An indentation made into the dough should remain as an indicator when the dough has risen sufficiently.
13. Bake bread loaf and rolls for 20-25 minutes.

*Instructor can select various flours for this exercise: bread; cake. When using whole wheat flour, use 1 1/2 cups all-purpose flour and 1/2 cup whole wheat flour.

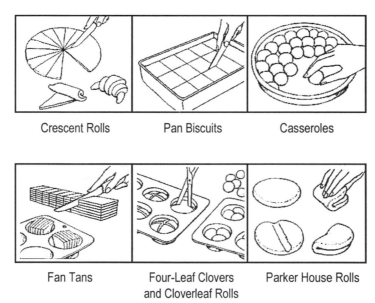

| Crescent Rolls | Pan Biscuits | Casseroles |

| Fan Tans | Four-Leaf Clovers and Cloverleaf Rolls | Parker House Rolls |

FIG3. Preparation of various dinner rolls. (Reprinted with permission of General Mills, Inc. *Betty Crocker's Cookbook*, copyright 1978, p. 213).

TABLE FOR EVALUATION OF YEAST BREAD			
Type of Flour	Height	Texture	Flavor

CHARACTERISTICS OF HIGH QUALITY YEAST BREADS

Volume: *High, well shaped loaf.*
Color: *Uniformly golden brown.*
Texture: *Even, no large air holes.*
Crumb: *Moist and silky, with an elastic quality.*

C. WATER BAGELS

1 package active dry yeast (do not use rapid rise)	1 1/2 teaspoons salt
1 cup warm water (105-115°F)	3 cups all-purpose flour
4 tablespoons sugar, divided	2 quarts water

1. Dissolve yeast in 1 cup water in large mixing bowl. Stir in sugar, salt, and 1 1/4 cups of the flour. Beat until smooth. Stir in remaining flour.
2. Turn dough onto lightly floured surface; knead until smooth and elastic, about 10 minutes. Place in greased bowl; turn grease side up. Cover; let rise in warm place until double, about 15 minutes. (Dough is ready if an indentation remains when touched.)
3. Punch dough down; divide into 6 or 8 (for bigger bagels, divide dough into 6 equal parts) equal parts. Roll each part into a rope 6 inches long; moisten ends with water and pinch to form a bagel. Let rise 20 minutes (start timing after first bagel is formed). Heat oven to 375°F.
4. In large kettle, heat 2 quarts of water to boiling. Add 2 tablespoons of sugar. Reduce heat; add 3-4 bagels, depending on the amount. Simmer 10 minutes, turning once. Drain on a kitchen towel. Bring water back to a boil. Repeat with remaining bagels. Bake on greased baking sheet until bagels are golden brown, 30-35 minutes; cool.

QUESTIONS

1. At what temperature should yeast be dissolved?

   What will happen if water is not hot enough or too hot?

2. Why should milk be scalded when used in a yeast dough recipe?

3.   What functional role does salt and sugar play in the fermentation process?

4.   a.   Discuss fermentation and the role of yeast in a yeast dough formula.

     b.   Give the formula for the fermentation process.

     c.   Name three types of yeast available to the consumer and what is the difference between them.

5.   What are the reasons for kneading?

6.   a.   What is "proofing" the dough?

     b.   What are the effects of over-proofing and under-proofing?

7.   a.   What is the difference between bread made from hard wheat flour and soft wheat flour?

     b.   Why?

8.   What happens when bread stales?

LABORATORY 5

Shortened- and Foam-Style Cakes

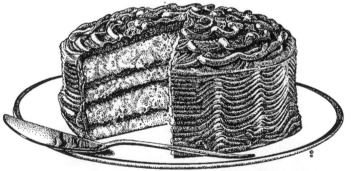

LABORATORY 5:
SHORTENED- AND FOAM-STYLE CAKES

Cake making is an art which requires exact measuring, mixing, and baking temperature. Shortened cakes contain fat, and today specialized fats have been developed that yield cakes that are superior in volume and texture, but not necessarily flavor. Foam-style cakes consist of sponge, angel food, and chiffon cakes and contain no added fat (except chiffon). The student will learn the proper techniques in cake making while learning the proper selection of ingredients and their functional roles.

VOCABULARY

angel food cake	emulsifier	plastic fat
chiffon cake	fold	soft peak stage (egg white foam)
creaming	Maillard browning	sponge cake
dry stage (egg white foam)	one bowl method	stiff peak stage (egg white foam)

OBJECTIVES

1. To learn the functional role of ingredients in shortened and foam-style cakes.
2. To learn the proper mixing and folding techniques when preparing shortened or foam-style cakes.
3. To identify the four stages of beating egg white foams for incorporation into foam-style cakes.
4. To demonstrate the effect of different pH levels in chocolate cake batters.

PRINCIPLES

1. Using the proper ingredients, measurements, and mixing techniques will insure a properly baked cake.
2. Sugar and fat contribute tenderness to a cake.
3. Plastic style fats incorporate air into a shortened cake batter which will contribute volume to a baked cake.
4. Creaming the fat and sugar will make a cake that is high in volume, fine in texture, and have better keeping quality (moist).
5. One-bowl method cakes require a plastic fat for complete incorporation, are lower in volume, and have poor keeping quality.
6. Foam-style cakes constitute:
   a. angel food cakes which are made with egg whites.
   b. sponge cake made with egg yolk and white.
   c. chiffon cake which is a cross between a foam-style cake and a shortened cake (contains oil).
7. The more egg whites are beaten, the more air is incorporated and the larger the volume of foam obtained. There are four stages of beating egg whites:
   a. _Foamy Stage_
      1. Egg white is lightly whipped and is frothy and fluid.
      2. It doesn't hold a peak. At this time add the salt, cream of tartar, and flavoring if specified in the recipe.
   b. _Soft Peak Stage_
      1. Foam appears white, moist, and shiny.
      2. It has small bubbles and flows in the bowl; peaks are formed but the tips of the peaks fold over. During the development of this stage, add sugar one tablespoon at a time if specified in the recipe.
   c. _Stiff Peak Stage_
      1. Foam does not flow in the bowl but is still shiny.
      2. When the beaters are removed, the peaks formed remain upright.
      3. A cut through the meringue leaves a clean path. **It is not advisable to whip egg whites beyond this stage.**
   d. _Dry Foam Stage_
      1. Egg whites achieve maximum volume and appear dry and curdled.
      2. When beaters are removed, foam breaks instead of forming peaks.
      3. Foam will collapse readily and is lumpy when added to other mixtures.
8. Baking pans for shortened cakes are greased and floured, while for foam-style cakes the pan is ungreased.

9. The pH of chocolate cake batters have an effect on the color of the cake: pH >7 the color is black while pH <7 a light brown color is the result. A cake with a pH=7 is mahogany red or "devil's food cake" color.

HIGH ALTITUDE ADJUSTMENTS

When baked above 3,000 feet, cakes will not rise properly. Use this chart as a guide when baking cakes at high altitudes. In addition, when baking a cake above 3,000 feet in altitude, increase the baking temperature by 25°F.

Ingredients	3,000 feet	5,000 feet	7,000 feet	10,000 feet
Sugar: for each cup, increase	1-3 teaspoons	1-2 tablespoons	1 1/2-3 tablespoons	2-3 1/2 tablespoons
Liquid: for each cup, add	1-2 tablespoons	2-4 tablespoons	3-4 tablespoons	3-4 tablespoons
Baking Powder: for each teaspoon, decrease	1/8 teaspoon	1/8-1/4 teaspoon	1/4 teaspoon	1/4-1/2 teaspoon

I. SHORTENED-STYLE CAKE

To evaluate cakes made by the creaming method and the one bowl method.

A. CREAMING METHOD

Butter-Style Cake

1/4 cup butter, margarine, or shortening*	1 cup cake flour
2/3 cup sugar	1 teaspoon baking powder
1/2 teaspoon vanilla extract	1/4 teaspoon salt
1 egg, beaten	1/3 cup milk

1. Preheat oven to 350°F. Set rack at middle position in the oven.
2. Cut waxed paper to fit the bottom of an 8-inch round cake pan.
3. Grease only the bottom of the cake pan; insert the waxed paper; grease the waxed paper.
4. Sift together the flour, salt, and baking powder; set aside.
5. Place the shortening and vanilla in the bowl. Set the mixer at medium speed. Add sugar very gradually. Cream until the mass is light and fluffy. The mass should be soft enough to remain on the bottom of the bowl; the mass should not be balled up around the mixer blades. Total creaming time may be as long as 5-7 minutes; this creaming step is critical.
6. Add the beaten egg in 2 portions. Beat for 1 minute after each addition.
7. Add approximately 1/3 of the flour mixture; beat for 1 minute. Add 1/2 of the milk and beat for 1 minute.
8. Add second portion of the flour mixture and liquid in the same manner as in step 7.
9. Add the last portion of the flour mixture. Beat batter for 1 minute.
10. Push all the batter at one time into the pan. Level batter with a rubber scraper. Bake for approximately 25 minutes.
11. Test cake for doneness by either touching the center of the cake with fingertip (it should spring back) or stick a toothpick in the center (it should come out clean).
12. Remove cake pan from oven and cool in an upright position for 10 minutes before removing. Let cake cool on a wire rack.

*Each unit should be assigned a specific fat. When the cakes are ready, each student should sample the finished product, and record the results in the table provided.

TABLE FOR EVALUATION OF SHORTENED CAKE MADE WITH CREAMING METHOD				
Fat	Crust Color	Grain	Moistness	Flavor
Butter				
Margarine				
Shortening				

CHARACTERISTICS OF A HIGH QUALITY BAKED CAKE

Color: Golden brown.
External Appearance: High with slightly rounded, smooth top.
Internal Appearance: Fine, even texture, not crumbly.
Body: Soft, velvety, slightly moist, light, tender.

QUESTIONS

1. a.   What role does the flour play in the cake?

    b.   How would you substitute all-purpose flour for the cake flour in the recipe?

2.   What role does sugar and fat play?

3. a.   Why would shortening cream better than butter or margarine?

    b.   Which cake would you prefer in flavor? Why?

4.   How is air incorporated into batters for shortened cakes?

5.   How is a shortened cake tested for doneness?

B. ONE BOWL METHOD

Butter-Type Cake

1 cup cake flour	1/4 cup shortening, butter, or margarine*
2/3 cup sugar	1/2 cup milk
1/4 teaspoon salt	1/2 teaspoon vanilla
1 1/2 teaspoons baking powder	1 egg

1. Preheat oven to 350°F. Set rack at middle position in the oven.
2. Cut waxed paper to fit bottom of an 8 inch round cake pan.
3. Grease only the bottom of the cake pan; insert the waxed paper; grease it again.
4. Sift together into a large mixing bowl the flour, sugar, salt, and baking powder.
5. Add the shortening, approximately half of the milk**, and the vanilla; **beat vigorously for 2 minutes**, scraping the bowl continuously. Use medium speed on the mixer.
6. Add unbeaten egg and remaining portion of milk. Beat two minutes longer using medium speed on electric mixer.
7. Push all the batter at one time into the cake pan. Level batter evenly. Bake for approximately 25 minutes.
8. Cool in upright position at least 10 minutes before removing from pan.

*Each unit should be assigned a specific fat. When the cakes are ready, each student should sample the finished product, and record the results in the table provided.
**If using all-purpose flour, add all the milk at this time.

TABLE FOR EVALUATION OF BUTTER TYPE CAKE - ONE BOWL METHOD				
Type of Fat	Crust Color	Grain	Moistness	Flavor
Butter				
Margarine				
Shortening				

QUESTION

1. How do cakes made with the one bowl method compare with cakes made with the creaming method?

FLAWS IN BAKED CAKES AND THEIR POSSIBLE CAUSES		
Flaw	Possible Causes	
Coarse Crumb Texture	Too much sugar Oven temperature too low	Not enough mixing after addition of flour
Cake High on Sides, Low in Center	Too much sugar, fat, leavening Not enough liquid Not enough mixing after addition of flour Too small pan for amount of batter	Oven temperature too low Cake was moved during baking Cake was not baked long enough
Heavy Compact Texture; Low Volume	Not enough leavening; gas lost before baking started Not enough air incorporated into creamed mixture Too much liquid, fat, or sugar	Too much mixing after addition of flour Pan too small for amount of batter Oven temperature too low
Lack of Tenderness; Dryness	Not enough fat, sugar, or liquid Too much flour or egg	Too much mixing after addition of flour
Sugary, Crispy Top	Too much sugar, fat, or leavening	
Humped, Cracked Top; Tunnels	Not enough fat and/or sugar Too much mixing after addition of flour	Too deep pan used for baking Oven temperature too high

46

II. TO DEMONSTRATE THE EFFECT OF CHANGING THE pH IN CHOCOLATE CAKE BATTERS

(A.) DEVIL'S FOOD CAKE

1 cup cake flour	1/4 cup shortening
3/4 cup sugar	1/2 cup buttermilk
3/4 teaspoon baking soda	1/2 teaspoon vanilla extract
1/2 teaspoon salt	1 egg
1/4 cup sifted cocoa	

1. Preheat oven to 375°F. Set rack on middle position in the oven.
2. Lightly grease bottom of 9 inch round cake pan. Insert waxed paper; lightly grease paper; evenly shake 1/2 teaspoon flour over bottom of pan.
3. Sift together cake flour, sugar, soda, salt, and cocoa.
4. Add vanilla to buttermilk; add buttermilk mixture and shortening to the dry ingredients.
5. Beat for 2 minutes using medium speed of mixer, scraping the sides of the bowl constantly.
6. Add unbeaten egg. Beat for 2 minutes, scraping the sides of the bowl constantly.
7. Remove 1 tablespoon of cake batter; add 1 tablespoon distilled water; mix. Take the pH: _____.
8. Use a rubber spatula to push all batter into prepared cake pan. Level batter in pan.
9. Bake for 30 minutes or until cake tests done.
10. Cool in upright position 10 minutes before removing from pan. **Cake is extremely tender; be careful when removing from pan.**

(B) VARIATION 2

Follow Devil's Food Cake Recipe, except:

Use: 1 1/4 teaspoons baking powder in place of the baking soda

(C.) VARIATION 3

Follow Devil's Food Cake Recipe, except:

Use: 1/2 cup whole milk, instead of buttermilk and increase the baking soda to 1 1/4 teaspoons

TABLE FOR EVALUATION OF DEVIL'S FOOD CAKE				
		Baked Product		
Liquid and Leavening Used	pH	Cell Size	Flavor	Color
Devils Food Cake				
Variation 2				
Variation 3				

QUESTIONS

1. How did the pH variations affect the color of the chocolate cake?

2. How was the crumb of the chocolate cake affected by:

    a.   increasing the pH?

    b.   decreasing the pH?

3. How was the flavor of the chocolate cake affected by:

    a.   increasing pH?

    b.   decreasing pH?

III. FOAM-STYLE CAKE

To learn and observe the stages that egg whites are to be whipped and the proper mixing and folding techniques to make a proper foam-style cake.

A. ANGEL FOOD CAKE

1 cup sifted cake flour	1 1/2 teaspoons cream of tartar
1 1/2 cups sugar	1 1/2 teaspoons vanilla extract
1/2 teaspoon salt	1/2 teaspoon almond extract
1 1/2 cups egg whites (about 12)	

1. Sift flour and salt together.
2. Beat the egg whites to the foamy stage.
3. Sprinkle cream of tartar and extracts over the foam and beat to the soft peak stage.
4. Add the sugar, 1 tablespoon at a time, until all the sugar is added. Egg whites should be at the stiff peak stage, but not dry.
5. Fold in approximately 1/4 of the flour and salt at a time, being careful to retain as much air as possible. Continue until you have added all flour mixture, carefully folding using a spatula (**do not use an electric mixer**).
6. Place in an **ungreased** 9 inch tube pan. Cut through the foam with a knife to distribute the batter evenly and to break up large air bubbles.
7. Bake on the bottom shelf in a preheated oven at 375°F for 40-45 minutes. Remove; invert cake and allow to cool thoroughly before removing from pan.

B. SPONGE CAKE

(Reprinted by permission of Southern Progress Corporation, *Cooking Light* Magazine, March/April, 1993, p. 67.)

1 cup cake flour	1 cup sugar, divided
1 teaspoon baking powder	2 teaspoons vanilla extract
1/4 teaspoon salt	1/4 cup water
3 eggs, separated	2 egg whites

1. Combine cake flour, baking powder, and salt; stir well, and set aside.

2. Beat 3 egg yolks in a large mixing bowl at high speed of an electric mixer for 1 minute.
3. Gradually add 3/4 cup sugar, beating constantly until egg yolks are thick and pale (about 5 minutes). Add vanilla and 1/4 cup water, beating at low speed until blended.
4. Add flour to egg yolk mixture, beating at low speed until blended; set aside.
5. Beat 5 egg whites (at room temperature) with an electric mixer until foamy. Gradually add remaining 1/4 cup sugar, 1 tablespoon at a time, beating until stiff peaks form.
6. Gently stir 1/4 of egg white mixture into batter. Gently fold in remaining egg white mixture.
7. Pour batter into an ungreased 9 inch tube pan. Bake at 375°F for 30-35 minutes or until cake springs back when touched lightly in center.
8. Invert pan; cool 60 minutes. Loosen cake from sides of pan using a narrow metal spatula; remove cake from pan.

C. JELLY ROLL CAKE (WHOLE EGG SPONGE CAKE)

3 large eggs, room temperature	1 teaspoon orange or lemon rind
1 cup sugar	1 teaspoon baking powder
1/3 cup water	1/4 teaspoon salt
1 teaspoon vanilla	1/2 cup confectioner's sugar
1 cup cake flour	3/4 cup strawberry preserves

1. Grease the bottom and sides of a jelly roll pan, 15 1/2 × 10 1/2 inches. Line the **bottom only** with aluminum foil. Grease the aluminum foil.
2. Preheat the oven to 375°F. Set rack on middle position in the oven.
3. Sift together flour, baking powder, and salt.
4. Beat eggs in a small (1 1/2 quart) mixing bowl, at high speed, for 5 minutes. Mixture must be thick and have tripled in bulk.
5. Place beaten eggs into a larger bowl (3 quart); gradually beat in the sugar.
6. Beat in water, vanilla, and orange rind on low speed.
7. Add dry ingredients in 3 portions; beating on low speed.
8. Pour the batter into the pan; level out the batter and then tap it lightly on the counter to remove excessive air bubbles.
9. Bake for 12-15 minutes or until top springs back when lightly touched with the finger.
10. Sift approximately 1/2 cup confectioner's sugar on a linen towel about the size of the pan.
11. Loosen edges of cake, turn out onto confectioner's sugar. Remove aluminum foil. Trim off any crusty edges or sides.
12. While cake is hot, start at narrow end and roll cake and towel together. Allow cake to cool in this position on a cooling rack.
13. When the cake is cold, carefully open towel and unroll. Carefully spread jelly on the cake, leaving 1 inch space on each end.
14. Carefully reroll the cake. Dust lightly with confectioner's sugar. Cut into 1 inch slices for serving.

TABLE FOR EVALUATION OF FOAM-TYPE CAKES					
		Baked Cake			
Cake	Appearance of Batter	Size	Grain	Texture	Flavor
Angel Food Cake					
Sponge Cake					
Jelly Roll Cake					

1. In making a sponge or angel food cake, what manipulative technique effects:

    a. large volume?

    b. a fine grain?

    c. a coarse texture?

2. What function does cream of tartar play in its addition to egg white foam?

3. Why is sugar added to the egg whites in the sponge and angel food cakes?

4. Why are foam cakes baked as soon as they are mixed?

5. What are the leavening agents in foam cakes?

6. What is the tenderizing agent in the angel food cake?

7. What role does cream of tartar play in the angel food cake?

8. What are the precautions of adding flour to egg white foams?

9. Discuss generally the nutrient composition of angel food, sponge, and shortened cakes?

LABORATORY 6

Pastry, Cream Puffs, and Popovers

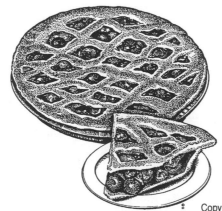

LABORATORY 6
PASTRY, CREAM PUFFS, AND POPOVERS

Pie dough is a simple product made up of flour, water, salt, and fat. The selection and manipulation of ingredients will have a strong effect on the tenderness and flakiness of the pie pastry. The leavening agent is steam which will contribute to flakiness. Steam is also responsible for the leavening effect observed in cream puffs and popovers. Therefore, the student will study pies, cream puffs, and popovers in this laboratory exercise and how manipulation of the ingredients and steam will affect the final quality.

VOCABULARY

cut in	pastry blender	plastic fat
flakiness	pastry method	tenderness
lard		

OBJECTIVES

1. To distinguish the difference between flakiness and tenderness in pastry dough.
2. To determine which fat contributes both tenderness and flakiness in a pastry dough.
3. To learn that proper manipulation will have a strong effect on the outcome of the pie dough, cream puffs, and popovers.
4. To observe how steam plays a common role in three different products: pastry, popovers, and cream puffs.

PRINCIPLES

1. The pastry method involves cutting the fat into the flour.
2. The type of fat used will determine the tenderness and flakiness of the pie crust.
3. Too much water and overmanipulation cause gluten to develop and will toughen the pie crust.
4. Steam is the leavening agent in pie crust, popovers, and cream puffs, therefore, a hot oven is needed.
5. Cream puffs are made with a unique mixing method that involves gelatinization of starch and addition of egg to provide structure and emulsification.

I. **TO LEARN AND OBSERVE HOW MANIPULATION AND STEAM WILL AFFECT CREAM PUFFS AND POPOVERS**

A. **CREAM PUFF SHELLS**

1/4 cup water
2 tablespoons butter or margarine
few grains salt

1/4 cup all-purpose flour
1 egg (well blended)

1. Preheat oven to 400°F.
2. Lightly grease three areas of a baking sheet, each area approximately 2 inches in diameter. Allow approximately 3 inches between greased areas.
3. Place water, butter, and salt in smallest size saucepan; heat until the butter is melted and water boils vigorously.
4. Add the flour all in one portion to the boiling water-fat mixture. Stir quickly with a wooden spoon to get flour well blended with the water-fat mixture. Stir mixture until it forms a ball. Cook for 1 minute over medium heat; remove saucepan from heat.
5. Partially cool the cooked starch paste.
6. Add the egg to the starch paste; stir vigorously to blend.
7. The starch paste should be sticky at this point. **If it has a greasy feel it is not correct. Beat another egg and add it to the paste a little at a time**. The mixture should be **sticky** at this point.

8. Divide paste mixture into approximately three equal portions. Place one portion on each of the greased areas of the baking sheet.
9. Bake for 35 minutes. Check after 25 minutes.
10. Remove shells from baking pan and cool on wire rack away from drafts. Fill with Creamy Vanilla Pudding.

B) CREAMY VANILLA PUDDING

1 1/2 cups skim milk
1/3 cup sugar
1/8 teaspoon salt
2 tablespoons cornstarch + 2 teaspoons

1 egg yolk
1 tablespoon margarine
1 1/2 teaspoons vanilla

1. Blend cornstarch, sugar, and salt in a 1 quart saucepan.
2. Mix together milk and egg yolk; add gradually to dry ingredients, dissolving any lumps if present.
3. Place saucepan over medium heat and stir constantly; bring to a boil and boil 1 minute; remove from heat.
4. Add margarine and vanilla; stir to incorporate ingredients.
5. Cool filling thoroughly before filling cream puffs. To prevent skin from forming on pudding place a piece of plastic wrap directly on the pudding's surface.

C) POPOVERS

1/2 cup all-purpose flour
1/4 teaspoon salt
1/2 cup milk

1 egg
vegetable oil to grease custard cups

1. Preheat oven to 450°F. Set rack to lowest position in oven.
2. Thoroughly grease bottom and sides of 3 or 4 custard cups, popover pans, or deep aluminum muffin tins.
3. Sift salt and flour together in a 1 quart mixing bowl.
4. Add egg to milk. Blend.
5. Gradually add egg-milk mixture to flour mixture and use a rotary beater to blend liquid and dry ingredients. Beat until mixture is smooth (to overbeat will reduce volume).
6.* Fill custard cups or popover pans 1/3-1/2 full. Muffin tins are to be 1/2 full.
7. If using custard cups, place on a baking sheet. Place in oven.
8. Bake for 20 minutes; reduce oven temperature to 350°F for 20 minutes more. **CAUTION**: Do not take popovers out too early or they will collapse.

*Hint: If using popover pans, preheat pans while preparing batter. This will help to create steam and bigger popovers.

TABLE FOR EVALUATION OF CREAM PUFFS AND POPOVERS				
Product	Observation of Batter	Crust Color	Flavor	Volume
Cream Puffs				
Popovers				

QUESTIONS

1. What is the difference between the appearance of cream puff dough and popover batter?

2. What is the difference in ingredients between cream puffs and popovers?

3. Would overmanipulation have an effect on these products?

4. What function does the egg perform in the cream puffs?

5. If the cream puff batter appears greasy after the egg has been added, how may you correct the situation? How should the dough look?

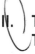

II. TO DETERMINE WHICH FAT CONTRIBUTES BOTH TENDERNESS AND FLAKINESS IN A PIE CRUST THROUGH PROPER MANIPULATION

A. PIE CRUST (BASIC RECIPE)

1 cup all purpose flour   1/3 cup shortening, butter, margarine, or lard
1/2 teaspoon salt   2-3 tablespoons cold water

1. Stir together flour and salt.
2. Cut fat into the flour until the mixture resembles cornmeal.
3. Sprinkle water and toss with a fork until flour adheres in large clumps.
4. Press dough into ball, using the tips of your fingers.
5. Cover dough with plastic wrap and refrigerate for 10 minutes. This allows for more hydration and also relaxes the dough to allow for easier rolling.

Rolling of Dough (*FIG.1*)

6. Place the dough between two sheets of wax paper for easier rolling.
7. Sprinkle the bottom sheet of waxed paper with flour. Take the dough, place it on the waxed paper, and slightly flatten it with the palm of your hand.
8. Place the second sheet of waxed paper on top. Place the rolling pin at the center of the mound of dough and start rolling from the center outward. This should be continued the entire time. **Never run the rolling pin back and forth over the dough as it will only toughen the pastry.**

    FIG.1. Roll the dough from the center outward
            to the edge.

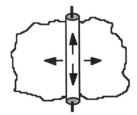

9. Loosen pastry dough from the waxed paper with minimum stretching of the pastry.
10. Ease the dough into the pie pan but be careful not to stretch the dough. Gently press the pastry dough against the bottom and sides of the pie pan. Trim the crust even with the edge of the pie pan.
11. If shell is going to be baked without a filling, prick the bottom and sides of the crust to allow steam to escape.
12. Bake at 450°F for 8-10 minutes or until pale golden brown.
Remember: (a) Crust will have a blistered effect: this is a sign of flakiness. (b) A light color is desirable; too dark will cause the fat to break down. (c) If the crust was not pricked sufficiently, puffing will occur because the steam was not allowed to escape.

B. LOW FAT PIE CRUST

1 1/4 cups all-purpose flour   1/4 cup shortening
1/4 teaspoon salt   4-5 tablespoons cold water

1.   Stir together flour and salt.
2.   Cut fat into the flour until the mixture resembles cornmeal.
3.   Sprinkle water over mixture and toss with a fork until flour adheres in large clumps.
4.   Press dough into a ball, using the tips of your fingers.
5.   Cover dough with plastic wrap and refrigerate for 10 minutes. This allows for more hydration and also relaxes the dough to allow easier rolling.
6.   Follow instruction from A.6. through A.12. concerning rolling and baking.

C. PIE CRUST WITH OIL

1 1/4 cups all-purpose flour   1/4 cup vegetable oil
1/4 teaspoon salt   1-2 tablespoons milk

1.   Mix together flour and salt in a bowl.
2.   Add oil and toss with a fork to combine.
3.   Add enough milk to hold dough together.
4.   Follow instructions from A.6. through A.12. concerning rolling and baking.

D.   PIE WAFERS

1.   Prepare Pie Crust (Basic Recipe) above, but each unit use a different fat. Allow pastry dough to rest 10 minutes before rolling.
2.   Cover the surface with waxed paper and place the pastry guides (1/4 inch thick) vertically and parallel to each other 4 inches apart on this covered surface.
3.   Place the dough between the pastry guides. Use your hands to pat out the dough into an oblong shape approximately 1 inch thick.
4.   Cover the dough with a sheet of waxed paper.
5.   Lightly roll the oblong-shaped dough with a rolling pin to obtain a uniform 1/4 inch thickness throughout the dough (*FIG.2*). **Be sure the product is not on the wood guides after shaping is completed. This is important so that the dough thickness is controlled**.
6.   Gently peel off the upper layer of waxed paper. Cut the pastry into uniform sized wafers (1 1/2 × 2 1/2 inches).
7.   Prick the wafers uniformly (with a fork in 3 places) to avoid blistering during baking.
8.   Bake at 450°F for approximately 8-10 minutes. Watch the time carefully and remove the wafers when a very light brown.
9.   Cool; place on racks to cool thoroughly. Evaluate the wafers for flakiness and tenderness.

FIG.2. Roll pastry between pastry guides to a uniform
          thickness of 1/4 inch.

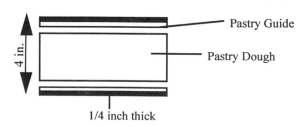

TABLE FOR EVALUATION OF PASTRY WAFERS				
Shortening Used	Blistering Effect	Flakiness*	Tenderness**	Flavor
Shortening				
Lard				
Butter				
Margarine				
Oil				

*Flakiness can be described as: 1. very thick layers; 2. moderately thick layers; 3. slightly thick/thin layers; 4. moderately thin layers; and 5. very thin layers.

**Tenderness can be described as: 1. very tough/crumbly; 2. moderately tough/crumbly; 3. slightly tough/crumbly; 4. tender; and 5. very tender.

CHARACTERISTICS OF HIGH QUALITY PIE PASTRY

Color: Light brown.
Appearance: Blistered on top.
Tenderness: Cuts easily and holds its shape.
Flakiness: Has layers that can separate easily.

QUESTIONS

1. a.   What shortening produced the tenderest crust? Why?

    b.   The flakiest crust? Why?

    c.   The flakiest and most tender crust? Why?

2. What effect would manipulation have on the final product?

3. Give some reasons which could cause a tough pie crust?

4. What effect would too much water have on the pie crust?

    Too little water?

5. a. Why is all-purpose flour used for pie crusts?

    b. Could you substitute cake flour and if so, how much?

6. Why is oil used at a lower rate than a solid fat in the pie crust recipe?

E. APPLE PIE

Pastry for 6 inch, 2 crust pie (double crust recipe)
3 medium size apples (Rome Beauty or any type of cooking apple)
2 tablespoons sugar
few grains salt

1 teaspoon cornstarch
1 teaspoon butter or margarine
1/8 teaspoon nutmeg
1/4 teaspoon cinnamon

1. Pare and slice apples into unbaked pie shell.
2. Add sugar, cornstarch, salt, butter, and spices.
3. Cover fruit with pastry topping.
4. Bake at 425°F for 30 minutes.

F. CREAM PIE FILLING

2 cups 1 1/2% milk
1/2 cup sugar
1/2 teaspoon salt
3 1/2 tablespoons cornstarch

1 egg yolk
2 teaspoons margarine
1 teaspoon vanilla
1 baked pie shell (6 inch)

1. Mix together sugar, salt, and cornstarch into saucepan.
2. Blend together milk and egg yolk. Add to dry ingredients from step 1.
3. Cook over medium heat. Stir constantly. When mixture boils, allow it to boil for 1 minute. Remove from heat.
4. Add margarine and vanilla. Stir until margarine is melted. Place filling in a bowl and place a piece of plastic wrap directly on the surface of the filling.
5. When cool, place filling into a baked pie shell.

Variations
a. Banana Cream Pie: Add 1 sliced banana to the baked pie shell before pouring in the cool filling.
b. Coconut Cream Pie: Add 1/3 cup grated sweetened coconut after removing the filling from the heat.
c. Chocolate Pie: Increase the sugar to 3/4 cup; add 1 1/2 squares unsweetened chocolate (shaved) to the milk and dry ingredients. Proceed as in the Basic Recipe (Cream Pie Filling).

G. LEMON MERINGUE PIE

1/2 cup sugar
2 1/2 tablespoons cornstarch
1/8 teaspoon salt
1 cup skim milk
2 eggs, separated

1/2 teaspoon lemon peel, grated
2 1/2 tablespoons lemon juice
2 teaspoons margarine or butter
1 baked pie shell (6 inch)

1. Combine sugar, cornstarch, and salt in a saucepan.

2. Mix together the **egg yolks** and the milk. Add to the dry ingredients and blend well, taking care to dissolve all lumps.
3. Cook over medium heat; stirring constantly; bring to a boil and allow to boil for 1 minute.
4. Remove from heat. Add lemon juice gradually. Add rind and margarine. Pour filling into baked pie shell.
5. Make meringue.

Meringue

2 egg whites   3 tablespoons sugar
1/4 teaspoon cream of tartar   1/4 teaspoon vanilla

1. Beat egg whites to the foamy stage; add cream of tartar and vanilla.
2. Beat until soft peaks are formed. Add sugar 1 tablespoon at a time. Beat until you can no longer feel the sugar between your fingers when you touch the meringue.
3. Place meringue on top of hot filling; make sure meringue touches the crust; this acts as a seal.
4. Bake at 350°F for 12-15 minutes.

H. QUICHE LORRAINE

Pastry for 9 inch one crust pie   2 egg whites or 1/2 cup egg substitute
6 slices turkey bacon, crisply cooked and crumbled   2 cups 1 1/2% milk
1 cup (4 ounces) natural Swiss cheese or Gruyere cheese, shredded   1/2 teaspoon salt
1/3 cup onion, finely chopped, cooked until softened   1/4 teaspoon black pepper
2 eggs   1/8 teaspoon ground red pepper

1. Heat oven to 425°F. Prepare pastry. Sprinkle cheese, bacon, and onion in pastry lined pie plate.
2. Beat eggs and egg whites slightly; beat in remaining ingredients. Pour into pie plate.
3. Bake for 15 minutes.
4. Reduce oven to 300°F. Bake until knife inserted in center comes out clean, about 30 minutes longer. Let stand 10 minutes before cutting.

I. CHICKEN POT PIE

1 package (10 ounces) frozen peas and carrots   1/4 teaspoon pepper
3 tablespoons margarine or butter   1 3/4 cups chicken broth (see recipe below)
1/3 cup all-purpose flour   2/3 cup skim milk
1/3 cup onion, chopped   2 1/2-3 cups chicken, cooked cut up
1/2 teaspoon salt   Pastry for 9 inch two crust pie (double crust recipe)

Broth

3 cups water   1/4 teaspoon thyme
1 large boneless chicken breast   3 chicken bouillon cubes
2 onions, peeled and sliced   dash salt
2 celery stalks   dash pepper

Place ingredients in a large saucepan. Bring to a boil; cover and simmer for one hour.

1. Rinse frozen peas and carrots under running cold water to separate; drain.
2. Heat margarine in a 2-quart saucepan over low heat until melted. Stir in onion, salt, and pepper. Cook until onion is translucent. Add flour and mix thoroughly.
3. Cook, stirring constantly, until mixture is bubbly; remove from heat. Stir in broth and milk. Heat to boiling, stirring constantly. Boil and stir 1 minute. Stir in chicken and vegetables.

4.   Pour filling into prepared crust; place other part of the crust over filling. Place slits at the top of the crust.
5.   Bake in a 425°F for about 30-35 minutes, or until sauce bubbles through slits. Cool 10 minutes before serving.

QUESTIONS

1.   Why are slits made in the top crust of a 2-crust pie?

2.   How can you prevent the edges of the pie crust from burning?

3.   Why is the lemon juice in the lemon meringue pie filling put in at the end of the cooking period?

4.   In all the cream fillings, sauces, etc., why is the mixture boiled for 1 minute?

5.   What type of pie pan is best for making pies?

6.   How can a pie be used as part of a meal?

LABORATORY 7

Fruit Selection and Cookery

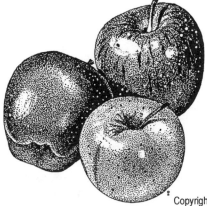

LABORATORY 7
FRUIT SELECTION AND COOKERY

There are many varieties of fruit that can be found in the market. This laboratory exercise is designed to demonstrate to the student how selection of a particular variety of fruit will affect its preparation.

VOCABULARY

antioxidant	osmosis	polyphenoloxidase
cellulose	pectic acid	rehydrate
dried fruit	pectin	semipermeable membrane
hemicellulose	protopectin	sulfur dioxide
modified atmospheric storage		

OBJECTIVES

1. To study the principle of osmosis and its effect on the structural properties of fruit during cooking.
2. To study the prevention of browning in fresh fruit through the use of antioxidants.
3. To observe the effect of moist or dry heat and sugar on cooked fruit.
4. To learn the proper way to rehydrate and cook dried fruit.
5. To emphasize that different varieties of the same fruit will not have the same cooking properties.

PRINCIPLES

1. Osmotic pressure causes:
   a. rupture of cell structure when fruit is cooked in water.
   b. retention of cell structure when fruit is cooked in syrup.
2. Fruit can be cooked in a variety of ways: poached, baked, broiled, sauteed; but not all varieties of the same kind of fruit can be cooked the same way.
3. The two pigments found in fruit are carotenoids and anthocyanins.
4. When certain fruits are cut, darkening takes place caused by enzymatic activity. Antioxidants are used to prevent this darkening.
5. During the ripening process, protopectin is changed to pectin, and this pectin in a certain amount can form a gel in the presence of the proper amount of sugar, water, and acid.

I. TO STUDY THE PREVENTION OF BROWNING IN FRESH FRUIT THROUGH THE USE OF ANTIOXIDANTS

A. BROWNING OF FRUIT

1. Slice a banana, pear, apple, or avocado and divide it into 6 lots.
2. Treat the 6 lots as indicated below.
   Treatment #1: Air.
   Treatment #2: Cream of Tartar solution (1/8 teaspoon to 1/2 cup water).
   Treatment #3: Lemon juice solution (1/8 teaspoon to 1/2 cup water).
   Treatment #4: Ascorbic acid solution (1/8 teaspoon to 1/2 cup water).
   Treatment #5: Salt solution (1/8 teaspoon to 1/2 cup water).
   Treatment #6: Blanch in boiling water 3 minutes.
3. Record any color change at the end of 30 minutes.

TABLE FOR EVALUATION OF FRUIT BROWNING			
Fruit	Treatment	Observation	Explanation
Banana	#1		
	#2		
	#3		
	#4		
	#5		
	#6		
Pear	#1		
	#2		
	#3		
	#4		
	#5		
	#6		
Apple (Red Delicious)	#1		
	#2		
	#3		
	#4		
	#5		
	#6		
Apple (Golden Delicious)	#1		
	#2		
	#3		
	#4		
	#5		
	#6		
Avocado	#1		
	#2		
	#3		
	#4		
	#5		
	#6		

<u>QUESTIONS</u>

1. Describe the process of enzymatic browning.

2. List ways enzymatic browning can be prevented and explain why each is effective.

3. Explain why fruits turn brown when bruised, even when the peel is intact.

4. Why is it that bananas mixed with cubed oranges in a fruit cup do not turn brown?

II. TO IDENTIFY THE FACTORS THAT INFLUENCE THE QUALITY OF COOKED APPLES

Select five cultivars of apples for each preparation.

A. ORANGE HONEY BAKED APPLE

1 large baking apple	dash nutmeg
1/4 cup orange juice	dash cinnamon
1 tablespoon honey	

1. Preheat oven to 375°F.
2. Rinse and core apple. Using a vegetable peeler, remove about a 1 inch strip of apple skin around center of apple.
3. Place apple in a 1 quart casserole.
4. Combine orange juice, honey, nutmeg, and cinnamon; stir to dissolve honey; pour over apple. Cover dish.
5. Bake apple for 25 minutes. Uncover and baste frequently with juice for an additional 20-25 minutes. Remove from oven. Cool slightly.

B. APPLESAUCE

2 medium apples	2 tablespoons sugar
1/2 cup boiling water	

1. Wash, peel, and quarter apples. Core each quarter and cut in 3-4 slices.
2. Add apple slices to boiling water; cover saucepan; simmer until slices are soft and tender, about 15-20 minutes.
3. Stir cooked apple slices with a fork until slices are broken up. Add sugar and stir until sugar is dissolved.

C. CODDLED APPLE

1 medium apple	3/4 cup water
1/2 cup sugar	

1. Add sugar to water in a wide bottom saucepan. Stir until sugar is dissolved. Bring to a boil. Remove from heat.
2. Wash, peel, core, and cut apple into 1/4 inch rings.
3. Add apples to hot syrup and cover saucepan. Reduce heat so apples cook slowly for about 20 minutes or until apple slices are translucent and clear.

TABLE FOR EVALUATION OF COOKED APPLES				
Variety	Cooking Style	Flavor	Texture	Appearance
	Sauce			
	Coddled			
	Baked			
	Sauce			
	Coddled			
	Baked			
	Sauce			
	Coddled			
	Baked			
	Sauce			
	Coddled			
	Baked			
	Sauce			
	Coddled			
	Baked			

QUESTIONS

1. Why does fruit soften when it is cooked in water?

2. Why are fruits cooked in syrup more translucent than when raw?

3. Explain the effect of the different concentrations of sugar on texture, shape, and fruit flavor.

III. TO OBSERVE FRUITS THAT HAVE ENOUGH PECTIN TO FORM A GEL WHEN SUGAR AND WATER ARE ADDED

A. CRANBERRY JELLY

1 cup cranberries   1/2 cup sugar
1/2 cup water

1. Sort and wash cranberries. Place in saucepan.
2. Add water. Bring to a boil; boil for 5 minutes or until the skin has popped open.

3. Rub the cooked berries through a strainer or put through a food mill, collecting the juice and as much of the pulp as possible in a clean saucepan placed underneath.
4. Add sugar to sieved pulp. Stir until sugar is dissolved.
5. Heat quickly to boiling temperature and boil for 5 minutes. Stir constantly to prevent mixture from sticking.
6. At the end of the cooking period, the mixture should be given a jelly "sheeting test": Several drops of juice tend to flow together from the side of the spoon (cook until the test is reached).
7. Pour into a serving dish. Do not stir this mixture as it cools.

QUESTIONS

1. During the ripening of fruit, follow the development of pectin; what enzymes are involved?

2. What are the ingredients needed for the setting of the pectin gel?

3. What acid is found in cranberries?

IV. TO OBSERVE THE VARIETY OF WAYS FRUITS CAN BE PREPARED

A. ORANGE POACHED PEARS

1/2 cup sugar
1/4 cup water
1/4 cup orange juice
6 whole cloves

1 tablespoon lemon juice
3 pears (Bartlett or Anjou)
Twist of orange rind (optional)

1. Combine sugar, water, orange juice, cloves, and lemon juice in a 2 quart saucepan; bring to a boil over medium heat, until sugar dissolves. Boil gently 5 minutes.
2. Peel pears and cut into chunks.
3. Add pears to the sugar syrup. Cover; reduce heat and simmer 15 minutes.
4. Transfer pears and syrup to a medium-sized bowl; remove cloves; cover and chill thoroughly.
5. Spoon pears and syrup into dessert dishes; top with a twist of orange rind if desired.

B. PRUNE-RAISIN BROWNIES

1/4 cup seedless raisins
3/4 cup pitted prunes
1 1/2 cups water, divided
1 1/2 cups cake flour
1 1/3 cups sugar
1 cup unsweetened cocoa
1 teaspoon instant coffee
2 teaspoons baking powder

1/2 teaspoon baking soda
1/2 teaspoon salt
1 large egg
2 large egg whites
2 tablespoons vegetable oil
2 teaspoons vanilla
3 tablespoons chopped walnuts

1. Position a rack in the center of the oven and preheat it to 350°F. Coat a 9 × 13 inch pan with cooking spray.
2. Combine the prunes and raisins with 1 cup of water in a saucepan, and bring to a boil. Lower the heat and simmer, covered, for about 5 minutes until soft. Remove from the heat and stir in the remaining 1/2 cup of water. Transfer to a food processor and puree. Set aside.

3. Sift together the flour, sugar, cocoa, instant coffee, baking powder, baking soda, and salt into a large bowl. Make a well in the center and add the egg and egg whites, oil, vanilla, and pureed fruit. With a whisk or an electric mixer on low speed, blend well.
4. Spread the batter evenly in the prepared pan and sprinkle on the chopped nuts. Bake for about 30-35 minutes, or until a tester in the center comes out clean; do not overbake. Cool on a wire rack; then cut into 24 brownies.

C. TROPICAL AMBROSIA

2 mangos, peeled and cut into bite-sized chunks
2 large navel oranges, peeled
2 bananas, peeled and thinly sliced
1 cup fresh pineapple, cut in thin wedges

1/2 honeydew melon, flesh cut into bite-sized chunks
1/3 cup confectioners sugar, sifted
1 can (3 1/2-ounces) flaked coconut
1/4 cup orange juice

1. Remove all outer white membrane from oranges and slice thin crosswise.
2. Layer oranges, bananas, mangos, honeydew, and pineapple in serving bowl, sprinkling with sugar, coconut, and orange juice as you go.
3. Cover and chill 2-3 hours. Mix lightly and serve.

D. BROILED GRAPEFRUIT

1 medium-size grapefruit, halved
4 teaspoons light brown sugar

1 tablespoon butter or margarine, melted

1. Preheat broiler.
2. Cut around grapefruit sections to loosen, then sprinkle each grapefruit half with 2 teaspoons brown sugar and drizzle with 1/2 tablespoon melted butter.
3. Broil 5 inches from heat 5-7 minutes until golden and serve hot.

Variations
1. Honey-Broiled Grapefruit: Substitute 1 tablespoon honey for each teaspoon of brown sugar and proceed as directed.
2. Broiled Oranges, Peaches, Apricots, Pears, or Pineapples: Halved oranges, peaches, apricots, and pineapple rings can be broiled. Sprinkle cut sides with light brown sugar and butter and broil 3-5 minutes until delicately browned.

E. BAKED APPLE CRUMBLE

Apple Layer:

2 cups each: Golden Delicious, Rome Beauty and Granny Smith, peeled and sliced
2 tablespoons orange juice
1/2 cup light brown sugar, firmly packed

1/3 cup all-purpose flour
3/4 teaspoon cinnamon
2 tablespoons margarine

Topping:

1/2 cup vanilla low-fat yogurt, divided

For apple layer:
1. Heat oven to 375°F. Spray a 2-quart casserole or baking dish with vegetable spray.
2. Arrange apples evenly in dish. Drizzle with orange juice.
3. Combine sugar, flour, and cinnamon. Mix in margarine until crumbly. Spoon over apples.
4. Bake at 375°F for 35 minutes or until apples are tender. Cool slightly. Serve warm.

For topping:
1. Spoon 1 tablespoon vanilla yogurt over each serving.

F.   APPLE-GINGERBREAD COBBLER

4 medium-sized cooking apples (such as Rome Beauty, Granny Smith), peeled and sliced
1 cup water
1/2 cup firmly packed brown sugar
1 tablespoon lemon juice
1/4 teaspoon ground cinnamon
2 teaspoons cornstarch
1 tablespoon water
1/2 cup buttermilk
1/4 cup sugar

1/4 cup unsulfured, mild flavored molasses
2 tablespoons vegetable oil
1 large egg
1/2 cup cake flour
1/2 cup whole wheat flour
1/2 teaspoon baking soda
1/2 teaspoon baking powder
1/4 teaspoon salt
1 teaspoon ground ginger
1/2 teaspoon ground cinnamon

1. Combine first 5 ingredients in a medium saucepan; stir well.
2. Bring to a boil; cover, reduce heat, and simmer 10 minutes or until apple is tender.
3. Combine cornstarch and 1 tablespoon water; add to apple mixture, stirring well.
4. Pour into a lightly greased 2 quart baking dish.
5. Combine buttermilk, 1/4 cup sugar, molasses, oil, and egg in a small mixing bowl; beat at medium speed with an electric mixer until smooth.
6. Combine cake and whole wheat flours with remaining ingredients; stir well.
7. Add to buttermilk mixture, beating until blended.
8. Pour batter over apple mixture.
9. Bake at 350°F for 35 minutes or until lightly browned. Serve warm.

GENERAL QUESTIONS

1. Why should fruit be boiled gently?

2. What effect does the degree of maturity have upon the quality of cooked apples?

3. Why are dried fruits sulfured?

4. What does the term tenderized mean on the label of dried fruit?

5. What are the principal nutritional contributions of fruits?

6. Why did the pears maintain their shape in the poaching recipe?

LABORATORY 8

Vegetables

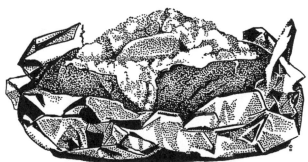

LABORATORY 8
VEGETABLES

Vegetables provide versatility and variety to a meal. When preparing vegetables the student must preserve the color, texture, and nutrients that are inherent to a particular vegetable. This laboratory exercise will introduce the student to the proper techniques of preparing vegetables as well as the use of vegetables for different parts of a meal.

VOCABULARY

anthocyanin
anthoxanthin
betalain

carotenoids
chlorophyll
chlorophyllin

flavonoids
pheophytin

OBJECTIVES

1. To learn how to recognize quality attributes in selecting fresh vegetables.
2. To learn how to maintain color, texture, flavor, and nutrients in the proper preparation of vegetables.
3. To recognize the versatility that vegetables contribute to the diet and to the meal.

PRINCIPLES

1. Vegetables come from different parts of a plant: leaf, stem, fruit, flower, root, tuber, bulb, and seed.
2. Vegetables can be cooked in a variety of ways: boiling, broiling, baking, steaming, frying, oven frying, stir frying (or panning), microwaving, or pressure cooking.
3. The main objective when cooking vegetables is to maintain color, texture, and nutritive value.
4. The color pigments in vegetables are categorized into
   a. chlorophyll: green
   b. carotenoids: yellow and orange; some red or pink
   c. anthocyanins: red, purple or blue
   d. anthoxanthins: white or colorless
   e. betalains: purplish red
5. Anthocyanins and anthoxanthins have many similarities in chemical structure, therefore, they are called flavonoid pigments.
6. In an alkaline medium, such as is provided by adding some soda to the cooking water:
   a. green color will intensify (chlorophyllin)
   b. no effect on carotenoids
   c. anthocyanins turn blue-green in color
   d. anthoxanthins turn yellow in color
   e. betalains turn brown in color
7. In an acid medium such as provided by adding lemon juice or cream of tartar to the cooking water:
   a. green color will turn olive green (pheophytin)
   b. no effect on carotenoids
   c. anthocyanins will become a reddish color
   d. anthoxanthins are bleached or colorless
   e. betalains will maintain color
8. The addition of an acid greatly retards the softening of cellulose making it extremely difficult to cook vegetables to the correct degree of doneness.
9. In an alkaline medium, the cellulose will soften very rapidly leading quickly to a very mushy texture as well as a loss of vitamins C and thiamin.
10. Boil vegetables whole and unpeeled whenever possible. The smaller the pieces, the greater the nutrient loss.

I. TO STUDY THE EFFECT OF HEAT AND pH ON PIGMENTS AND TEXTURE IN VEGETABLES

PROCEDURE

1. Place 1 cup water in each of four 1 quart saucepans.
2. Place the amount of alkaline or acid into respective saucepan as indicated in the chart.
3. Place small amount of vegetable in each saucepan.
4. Cook over low heat, covered, the amount of time as indicated.
5. Place vegetable on a white plate.
6. Place cooking liquid into a small custard cup.
7. Mark the table with your observations.

TABLE FOR EVALUATION OF VEGETABLES						
			Color and Texture			
Pigment	Color	Vegetable	1/4 teaspoon baking soda; 15 minutes	1/2 teaspoon cream of tartar; 15 minutes	15 minutes	30 minutes
Chlorophyll	Green	Broccoli				
Betalains	Red-Purple	Beets				
Anthoxanthins	Colorless	Onions				
Carotenoids	Yellow; Orange	Carrots				
Anthocyanins	Red-Blue	Red Cabbage				

QUESTIONS

1. What effect did the baking soda have on:

   a. carotenoids?

   b. betalains?

   c. anthocyanins?

   d. anthoxanthins?

   e. chlorophyll?

   f. texture of each vegetable?

2. What effect did the cream of tartar have on:

   a. carotenoids?

   b. betalains?

   c. anthocyanins?

   d. anthoxanthins?

   e. chlorophyll?

   f. texture of each vegetable?

3. What effect did prolonged moist heat have on maintaining texture and pigmentation?

4. What recommendations would you give?

II. TO PREPARE VEGETABLES IN A VARIETY OF WAYS AND TO RECOGNIZE QUALITY PARAMETERS IN SELECTION AND PREPARATION

A. PREPARATION OF MEALY AND WAXY POTATOES BY CONVENTIONAL BAKING AND MICROWAVE METHODS

Potatoes of different varieties are available in various parts of the country. Basically, potatoes can be classified as mealy or waxy. Usually potatoes that are round in shape will tend to be waxy, whereas the long flat ones tend to be starchy. Mealy potatoes are preferred for mashing, baking, and frying. Waxy potatoes are a good choice for boiling or in recipes requiring the potato to hold its shape (salads, stews).

1. Baked Potatoes - Oven Method

1. Preheat oven to 400°F.
2. Select a baking potato, a red potato, and an all-purpose potato.
3. Place washed, dried potatoes on a shallow baking pan. Do not crowd potatoes on the baking pan. Prick several places with a fork.

4. Bake until potatoes can be pierced easily with a fork. Medium sized potatoes in a 400°F oven may require 1-1 1/2 hours to bake. **Note**: If skins are to be eaten, a small amount of fat can be rubbed over the surface of the potato skin to give a more tender skin on the baked potato.
5. As soon as potatoes are removed from the oven, the potatoes should be split open to allow steam to escape and prevent the potatoes from becoming soggy.

2. **Baked Potatoes - Microwave Method**

1. Select a baking potato, a red potato, and an all-purpose potato.
2. For whole potatoes, scrub oval potatoes (rather than long shapes) of similar size.
3. Pierce potatoes to allow steam to escape.
4. Arrange potatoes about 2 inches apart in circle in microwave (*FIG.1*). (If potatoes are old, long, or dry, wrap each in waxed paper before placing in microwave. For crisper skins, sprinkle dampened potatoes with salt.)
5. Microwave potatoes uncovered on high (100%) until tender, 11-13 minutes. Let stand 5 minutes. (Potatoes hold their heat well; if microwaving a second vegetable, cook potatoes first.)

Watch time

FIG.1. Arrange potatoes about 2 inches apart in circle in microwave. (Reprinted with the permission of General Mills, Inc. *Betty Crocker's Microwave Cookbook*, Random House, Inc., 1981).

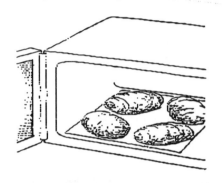

TABLE FOR EVALUATION OF BAKED POTATOES				
Variety	Method	Appearance	Flavor	Moistness and Texture
Baking Potato	Conventional			
Red Potato	Conventional			
All-Purpose Potato	Conventional			
Baking Potato	Microwaved			
Red Potato	Microwaved			
All-Purpose Potato	Microwaved			

CHARACTERISTICS OF HIGH QUALITY BAKED WHITE POTATOES

Appearance: *White, opaque, or slightly translucent depending on varieties.*
Texture: *Cell structure is pliable, mealy, light.*
Moistness: *Dry.*
Flavor: *Bland, yet slightly sweet.*

B. COMPARISON OF TWO COOKING METHODS FOR BROCCOLI: STEAMING VS. MICROWAVE

1. Broccoli: Steaming Method

1. Place 1-2 inches of water in a two-quart saucepan. Enough water must be used to produce steam for entire cooking time.
2. Place cleaned broccoli, cut into flowerets, into steamer basket; position over water. Tightly cover pan.
3. Bring water quickly to boiling over high heat. When water is boiling, reduce heat to keep water boiling slowly.
4. Cook broccoli approximately 5-7 minutes. Test with a fork until tender.

2. Broccoli: Microwave Method

1. Trim off large leaves; remove tough ends of lower stems; wash broccoli.
2. For spears, cut broccoli lengthwise into thin stalks. If stems are thicker than 1 inch, make lengthwise gashes in each stem.
3. Place 1/4 cup water and 1/8 teaspoon salt in baking dish, 12 × 7 1/2 × 2 inches, or 10 inch pie plate.
4. Arrange broccoli stalks in baking dish (tips in center) (*FIG.2*) or arrange in circle in 10 inch pie plate with tips in center of plate.
5. Cover with plastic wrap and microwave on high (100%) for 4 minutes; rotate baking dish or pie plate 1/2 turn.
6. Microwave until tender, 3-5 minutes longer; drain.

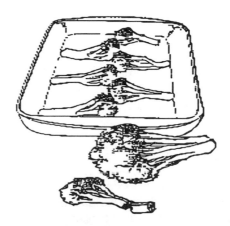

FIG.2. Arrange broccoli stalks in baking dish (tips in center). (Reprinted with the permission of General Mills, Inc. *Betty Crocker's Microwave Cookbook*, Random House, Inc., 1981).

TABLE FOR EVALUATION OF BROCCOLI			
Preparation Method	Color	Texture	Flavor
Steaming			
Microwaving			

Cheese Sauce For Broccoli (optional)

1 cup milk
2 tablespoons butter or margarine
2 tablespoons flour

1/4 teaspoon salt
1 cup mild Cheddar cheese, grated

1. Melt butter in a saucepan; add flour and salt; blend.
2. Remove from heat; add milk in portions; stir after each addition to form a smooth paste.
3. Bring to a boil over direct heat; boil 1 minute, stirring.
4. Remove from heat. Add cheese. Stir until well blended.
5. Place the hot cooked vegetable in warm dish. Pour hot sauce over vegetable. **Use only sufficient sauce to cover; do not drown the vegetable in sauce.**

1. When cooking broccoli, which method produced the best color? Why?

2. For potatoes, which method would you recommend: conventional or microwave?

3. Why is there a tendency to overcook potatoes in a microwave? What is meant by standing time?

4. What is the advantage of using the microwave? What is the disadvantage of using the microwave?

5. What factors would affect cooking time for a vegetable?

III. VEGETABLE PREPARATION

Vegetables can be used for different parts of a meal. This section illustrates how vegetables can serve as a main course as well as an accompaniment to the meal. Baking, steaming, and stir frying have been cited as conservatory methods for cooking vegetables. Another method, "oven-fry" will be used to lower fat content, but still retain the quality of the prepared dish.

A. MINESTRONE SOUP

1 can (10 ounces) red kidney beans
1 large yellow onion, peeled and minced
1 clove garlic, peeled and minced
3 slices turkey bacon, minced
1 tablespoon vegetable oil
1 1/2 quarts beef broth or 1/2 and 1/2 mixture of water and beef broth
    (6 cups water + 3 bouillon cubes)
2 medium size carrots, peeled and diced
1 medium potato, peeled and diced
1 cup cabbage, finely shredded

1/4 cup celery, minced
2 1/2 tablespoons tomato paste
1/2 teaspoon dried basil
1/4 teaspoon oregano
1/8 teaspoon thyme
1 teaspoon salt
1/8 teaspoon pepper
1/2 tablespoon parsley, minced
1/2 cup ditalini or elbow macaroni
2 1/2 tablespoons Parmesan cheese

1. Stir-fry onion, garlic, and bacon in oil in a large, heavy kettle (5-8 minutes) over moderate heat until onion is pale golden.
2. Add broth and all the remaining ingredients except parsley, pasta, and Parmesan; cover; simmer for 1 hour, stirring now and then.
3. Add parsley and pasta; cover and simmer 15-20 minutes longer until pasta is tender.
4. Taste for salt and adjust as needed. Stir Parmesan into soup or if you prefer, pass it separately.

B. STUFFED TOMATOES

4 large, firm, ripe tomatoes, washed
1/2 teaspoon salt
1/8 teaspoon pepper

Stuffing

1 tablespoon butter or margarine
1/4 cup yellow onion, finely chopped
1 clove garlic, finely chopped
2 cups soft bread crumbs
2 tablespoons parsley, finely chopped
1/2 teaspoon oregano
3/4 teaspoon salt
1/8 teaspoon pepper
1 cup tomato pulp (saved from tomato centers), chopped
1/4 cup Parmesan cheese, grated

1. Heat oven to 375°F.
2. Cut a thin slice from the top of each tomato.
3. Using a teaspoon, scoop out pulp and seeds; coarse chop pulp and reserve 1 cup (use rest in soup or stew).
4. Sprinkle inside with salt and pepper.
5. Melt butter in a small skillet over moderate heat, add onion and garlic; saute 8-10 minutes until golden.
6. Mix onion and garlic with remaining stuffing ingredients except Parmesan and oregano.
7. Stuff tomatoes, sprinkle with Parmesan and oregano. Stand tomatoes in a buttered shallow casserole and bake uncovered, 1/2 hour or until tender.

C. SWEET-SOUR RED CABBAGE

1 medium onion, sliced
1 teaspoon dry mustard
1 tablespoon margarine
1 pound red cabbage, finely shredded
2 tart, medium apples, sliced
2 tablespoons brown sugar

1 tablespoon Dijon mustard
3 tablespoons balsamic vinegar
1/2 cup water
1/2 teaspoon salt or to taste
1/4 teaspoon ground pepper

1. Heat margarine in large skillet. Add onion and dry mustard. Cook until onion is tender.
2. Add apple slices and brown sugar; cook 5 minutes.
3. Add cabbage, Dijon mustard, vinegar, water, and seasonings.
4. Bring mixture to a boil; lower heat and cover.
5. Cook over low heat for approximately 45 minutes or until cabbage is tender. Stir often.

D. CAULIFLOWER AU GRATIN

1 large cauliflower, divided into flowerets, boiled and
    drained
1/2 teaspoon salt
1/8 teaspoon white pepper

1 1/2 cups hot cheese sauce (See Cheese Sauce for
    Broccoli)
1/3 cup sharp Cheddar cheese, coarsely grated
1 tablespoon butter or margarine, melted

1. Preheat broiler.
2. Arrange flowerets in an ungreased au gratin dish or shallow casserole.
3. Season with salt and pepper and cover evenly with sauce.
4. Sprinkle with cheese and drizzle with butter.
5. Broil 5 inches from heat 3-4 minutes until cheese melts and is dappled with brown.

E. RATATOUILLE

1 medium eggplant, peeled, cut in 1/4 inch cubes
2 medium zucchini, sliced
2 teaspoons salt
1/4 cup olive oil
2 medium yellow onions, peeled and sliced thin
1 medium green pepper, cut into julienne strips
1 medium red pepper, cut into julienne strips

2 garlic cloves, peeled and crushed
2 medium tomatoes, coarsely chopped
1/4 teaspoon pepper
1 teaspoon garlic salt
1/2 teaspoon dried Italian seasoning
2 tablespoon minced parsley
2 cups frozen whole kernel corn, thawed

1. Cut eggplant in 1/4 inch cubes and stir fry, about 1/4 at a time, 3-5 minutes in 2-3 tablespoons oil over moderately high heat. Drain on paper towel (eggplant soaks up oil, but don't use more than 2-3 tablespoons for each batch or the ratatouille will be greasy).
2. Brown all zucchini in 2 tablespoons oil; drain.
3. Stir fry onions, garlic, green and red peppers in remaining oil over moderate heat for 10 minutes; lay tomatoes on top; add garlic salt, pepper, and Italian seasoning; cover and simmer 8-10 minutes; add corn.
4. Uncover and simmer 10 minutes longer.
5. In an ungreased shallow 2 1/2 quart flameproof casserole, build up alternate layers as follows: onion/pepper mixture, eggplant/zucchini (sprinkle with salt), onion/pepper mixture, eggplant/zucchini (sprinkle with salt), and onion/pepper mixture.
6. Simmer, covered, over low heat (do not stir) 30 minutes; uncover, simmer 20 minutes longer.

F. FETTUCINI PRIMAVERA

1 package (1 pound) fettucini

Vegetables
1 tablespoon butter or margarine
2 tablespoons salad oil
1 garlic clove, split
1 zucchini, sliced 1/4 inch thick
1/2 pound broccoli, cut into 1 1/2 inch flowerets
1/2 red pepper, cut into 1/4 inch strips
1/2 pound whole fresh snow pea pods, ends trimmed
4 ounces mushrooms, sliced

Sauce
2 tablespoons butter or margarine
1 cup 2% milk
1 cup Parmesan cheese, grated
1/4 teaspoon salt
dash pepper

2 tomatoes, peeled and chopped

1. Start cooking fettucini as package label directs.
2. **Prepare vegetables**:
    1. In 1 tablespoon hot butter and oil toss garlic, zucchini, broccoli, and red pepper; stir fry 5 minutes or until vegetables are just crisp.
    2. Add pea pods and mushrooms; cook 1 minute.
    3. Cook vegetables, covered, 1-2 minutes.
    4. Do not overcook. Discard garlic.
3. **Make sauce**:
    1. In medium saucepan, heat butter and 2% milk until butter is melted.
    2. Remove from heat. Add 3/4 cup cheese, salt, and pepper; mix well.
4. **Drain fettucini**:
    1. Toss with sauce; turn out onto heated serving platter.
    2. Place vegetables on top.
    3. Arrange tomatoes around edge.
    4. Sprinkle with 1/4 cup Parmesan cheese. Toss at table just before serving.

G. MOUSSAKA

Meat Sauce
1/2 cup onion, finely chopped
3/4 pound ground beef or lamb
1 garlic clove, crushed
1/4 teaspoon dried oregano leaves
1/2 teaspoon dried basil leaves
1/4 teaspoon ground cinnamon
1/2 teaspoon salt
dash of pepper
1 can (8 ounces) tomato sauce

Cream Sauce
1 tablespoon flour
1/4 teaspoon salt
dash of pepper
1 cup skim milk
1 egg

1 eggplant (about 1 1/2 pounds), washed
  and dried
salt
1/2 cup margarine melted

1/4 cup Parmesan cheese, grated
3/4 cup Cheddar cheese, grated
1 tablespoon dried bread crumbs

1. **Make meat sauce:**
    1. In a large saucepan, add chopped meat and brown over moderate heat; add onion and garlic and continue cooking, stirring occasionally until onion is soft
    2. Add oregano, basil, cinnamon, salt, pepper, and tomato sauce; bring to a boil, stirring. Reduce heat; simmer, uncovered, 1/2 hour.
2. **Broil eggplant:**
    1. Halve unpeeled eggplant lengthwise; cut crosswise into 1/2 inch thick slices. Place in bottom of broiler pan.
    2. Sprinkle lightly with salt; brush lightly with melted margarine. Broil 4 inches from heat, 4 minutes on each side, or until golden.
3. **Make cream sauce:**
    1. In medium saucepan, stir together flour, salt, and pepper. Add milk gradually.
    2. Bring to a boil, stirring until mixture is thickened. Remove from heat.
    3. In a small bowl, beat egg thoroughly. Beat in some of the hot cream-sauce mixture.
    4. Return mixture to saucepan; mix well.
4. **Assemble casserole:**
    1. In the bottom of a 9 × 9 × 2 inch square pan layer half of the eggplant overlapping slightly.
    2. Sprinkle with 1 tablespoon of Parmesan and Cheddar cheeses.
    3. Stir bread crumbs into meat sauce; spoon evenly over eggplant in casserole.
    4. Sprinkle with 1 tablespoon each Parmesan and Cheddar cheeses.
    5. Layer rest of eggplant, overlapping as before.
    6. Pour cream sauce over all. Sprinkle with any remaining cheese.
5. Bake at 350°F 35-40 minutes or until golden brown and top set.

H. SPAGHETTI SQUASH - ~~BAKED~~ *Microwave*

1 (2 pound) spaghetti squash, halved and seeded
1/4 teaspoon salt
2 cups prepared spaghetti sauce, heated

dash pepper
2 tablespoons butter or margarine
grated Parmesan cheese

1. Cut spaghetti squash in half and place in a large pot of boiling water.
2. Boil for 5 minutes.
3. Preheat oven to 375°F. Place each piece of squash, hollow side up, on a square piece of foil large enough to wrap it.
4. Sprinkle with salt and pepper and dot with butter. **Wrap** tightly.
5. Place squash on a baking sheet and bake 45 minutes until fork tender.
6. Unwrap and then, with a fork, scrape flesh into strands (*FIG.3*). Toss with Tomato Sauce and grated Parmesan cheese and place back into shell.

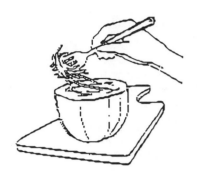

FIG.3. Scrape flesh into strands with a fork (Reprinted with the permission of General Mills, Inc. *Betty Crocker's Microwave Cookbook,* Random House, Inc., 1981).

I. ZUCCHINI LASAGNA

2 teaspoons olive oil
1 medium-size yellow onion, chopped (1 cup)
2 teaspoons minced garlic (4 cloves)
4 cans (8 ounces each) tomato sauce
1 cup sliced mushrooms
1 tablespoon dried basil, crumbled
5 medium-size zucchini (1 3/4 pounds), sliced lengthwise,
    1/4 inch thick

2 large egg whites, lightly beaten
1/4 cup plain dry bread crumbs
1/8 teaspoon black pepper, or to taste
1/2 teaspoon garlic salt
1 1/2 cups (12 ounces) part-skim ricotta cheese
1/4 cup minced leaf parsley
1/4 cup Romano cheese
3/4 cup shredded part-skim mozzarella cheese

1. In a large, heavy saucepan, heat the olive oil over moderate heat.
2. Add the onion, garlic, and mushrooms and sauté for 5 minutes or until soft.
3. Add the tomato sauce and basil and bring to a boil.
4. Lower the heat and simmer, stirring occasionally for 20 minutes or until the sauce has thickened and reduced to about 3 cups.
5. Remove from the heat and set aside.
6. Preheat the oven to 425°F.
7. Line a baking sheet with aluminum foil.
8. Place the zucchini slices in a single layer on the baking sheet. Brush the top sides with the 1 egg white, then sprinkle the bread crumbs, garlic salt, and pepper evenly over the slices.
9. Bake for 20 minutes or until the zucchini is golden and crisp tender when pierced with a knife.
10. Remove from the oven and set aside until cool enough to handle.
11. Reduce oven temperature to 350°F.
12. In a medium-size bowl, combine the ricotta cheese, egg white, parsley, and three tablespoons of the Romano cheese.
13. Grease an 11 × 7 × 2 inch baking dish.
14. Spread 1 cup of the tomato basil sauce evenly in the dish.
15. Arrange half of the zucchini on top of the sauce in a single layer, trimming the slices to fit if necessary.
16. Spread the ricotta-Romano mixture over the zucchini.
17. Sprinkle 1/4 cup of the mozzarella cheese over the top; spoon 3/4 cup sauce over the mozzarella.
18. Place the remaining zucchini in a single layer on top again, trimming to fit.
19. Spread the remaining 1 1/4 cups sauce evenly over the zucchini layer, then scatter the remaining 1/2 cup mozzarella cheese and 1 tablespoon Romano cheese over the sauce.
20. Place the dish on a baking sheet in case the lasagna bubbles over.
21. Bake for 35-45 minutes or until the cheese bubbles and the lasagna is hot in the center.
22. Cover the pan loosely with foil if the top browns too quickly.
23. Remove from the oven and let stand for 15 minutes before cutting into rectangles.

J. EGGPLANT PARMIGIANA

6 tablespoons all-purpose flour
1/4 cup toasted wheat germ
3 tablespoons sesame seeds
1/4 teaspoon salt
2 large egg whites
1 tablespoon water
1 large eggplant (1 pound), peeled, sliced 1/4 inch" thick
2 tablespoons olive oil

Herb Tomato Sauce
1 teaspoon olive oil
1/2 cup chopped onion
2 cans (8 ounces each) tomato sauce
1/4 teaspoon dried basil, crumbled
1/4 teaspoon dried oregano, crumbled
1/4 teaspoon salt
1/4 teaspoon pepper
1 1/2 teaspoon parsley

1 1/2 cups shredded part-skim mozzarella cheese

1. Prepare sauce and let simmer while fixing the eggplant.
   a. In a medium-size heavy saucepan, heat the oil over moderate heat.
   b. Add the onion and saute, stirring occasionally, for 5 minutes or until soft.
   c. Lower the heat and add tomato sauce, dried basil and oregano, salt, and pepper and bring to a simmer.
   d. Cook, covered, stirring occasionally, for 15 minutes.
   e. Stir in the parsley.
2. Preheat oven to 450°F.
3. Lightly grease a baking sheet.
4. On a large plate, combine the flour, wheat germ, sesame seeds, and salt.
5. In a shallow bowl, stir together the egg whites and water.
6. Dip the eggplant slices first in the egg white mixture, then in the flour mixture to coat.
7. Arrange on the baking sheet; drizzle each slice with the oil and bake for 10 minutes.
8. Lower the oven temperature to 400°F and bake 10 minutes longer.
9. Turn the eggplant slices over and bake another 10 minutes or until crisp, golden and tender.
10. Place eggplant in a lightly greased 9 × 11 × 2 inch pan.
11. Pour sauce over eggplant, then sprinkle with 1 1/2 cups shredded part-skim mozzarella cheese.
12. Bake 15-20 minutes until cheese has melted.

QUESTIONS

1. Why should water be boiling when the vegetables are added?

2. If the chief aim is to preserve color, how should these vegetables be cooked?

   a. beets

   b. broccoli

   c. carrots

d.   cauliflower

e.   spinach

f.   potatoes

3.   What are the advantages of cooking vegetables by panning?

LABORATORY 9

Salads

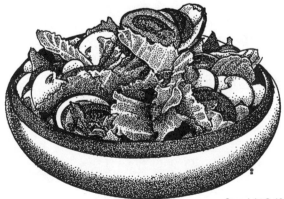

LABORATORY 9
SALADS

Cold, clean, crisp, and dry are the descriptive words for salad preparation. A salad adds color and texture to a meal, therefore, the proper selection and combination of ingredients are important. The student will learn the proper care of salad ingredients as well as the preparation of an attractive and palatable product that will enhance a meal.

VOCABULARY

accompaniment salad	dessert salad	main course salad
appetizer salad	garnish	salad greens

OBJECTIVES

1. To observe the proper preparation of salad greens.
2. To learn how color plays an important role in creating a salad.
3. To learn how flavor and texture balance is important in a salad.

PRINCIPLES

1. Salad greens must be washed and dried thoroughly before use.
2. Lukewarm water will open up crinkly-type leaves (such as spinach).
3. Green leaves should be torn and not cut into bite-size pieces.
4. A salad green should not be cut up so small that it will lose its identity.
5. Color and texture contrasts are important when creating a salad.
6. The dressing for the salad must be added right before it is served.
7. There are four types of salads:
   a. appetizer: whets the appetite.
   b. accompaniment: complements the meal.
   c. main dish salad: contains protein in the form of chicken, fish, cheese, etc.
   d. dessert salad: served at the end of the meal.

I.   APPETIZER SALAD

A.   ANTIPASTO SALAD PLATTER (APPETIZER)

2 medium red* peppers	1/2 teaspoon salt
2 tablespoons olive oil	1 garlic clove

*May use a combination of green and red peppers for more color.

1. Preheat oven to 450°F.
2. Wash peppers; drain well.
3. Place peppers on cookie sheet; bake about 20 minutes, until skin becomes blistered and charred. With tongs, turn peppers every 5 minutes.
4. Place hot peppers in large saucepan. Cover and let stand 15 minutes.
5. Peel off charred skin with sharp knife. Cut each pepper into fourths. Remove ribs and seeds; cut out any dark spots.
6. In bowl combine oil and other ingredients; add peppers and toss lightly to coat. Refrigerate.

Deviled Eggs

4 eggs
2 tablespoons mayonnaise

1/2 teaspoon dry mustard
1/8 teaspoon salt

1. Bring eggs to a boil; lower temperature and simmer for 10 minutes. Cool, peel, and cut lengthwise.
2. Scoop out yolk; mash and mix with mayonnaise, mustard, and salt.
3. Replace yolk mixture into egg white shell; refrigerate.

Assembly

1/4 pound hard Genoa salami
1/4 pound boiled ham

1/2 cup black olives, pitted

1. Roll up salami and ham; place alternately on round plate.
2. Place roasted peppers in center of plate. Place deviled eggs around the plate. Place olives on plate.

II. DINNER ACCOMPANIMENT SALADS

A. SPINACH-MUSHROOM SALAD

2 tablespoons vegetable oil
2 tablespoons wine vinegar or balsamic vinegar
1/4 teaspoon salt
generous dash of freshly ground black pepper
1 garlic clove, crushed

1 pound spinach, torn into bite-size pieces (about 8 cups)
8 ounces fresh mushrooms, sliced (about 3 cups)
2 slices turkey bacon, crisply cooked and crumbled
1 hard-cooked egg, chopped

1. Shake oil, vinegar, salt, pepper, and garlic in tightly covered container.
2. Toss with spinach and mushrooms.
3. Sprinkle with bacon and egg.

B. TOSSED GREEN SALAD WITH CHEESE MUSTARD DRESSING

4 slices of white bread, cubed
2 large garlic cloves, cut lengthwise into halves
2 tablespoons olive or vegetable oil
4 ouncesfresh mushrooms, sliced (about 1 1/2 cups)

1/2 head Boston lettuce, torn into bite-size pieces
1/2 small bunch Romaine, torn into bite-size pieces
Parmesan cheese

1. Prepare Cheese-Mustard Dressing (below).
2. Cut bread into cubes about 1 inch square. Cook and stir garlic in oil in 8 inch skillet over medium heat until garlic is deep golden brown; remove garlic and discard.
3. Add bread to oil. Cook and stir until bread is golden brown and crusty; cool.
4. Shake Cheese-Mustard Dressing; toss with mushrooms, Boston lettuce, and Romaine. Sprinkle with bread cubes and some Parmesan cheese.

Cheese-Mustard Dressing

2 tablespoons olive or vegetable oil
1 tablespoon red wine vinegar
2 teaspoons Parmesan cheese, grated
2 teaspoons Dijon-style mustard

1/4 teaspoon salt
1/4 teaspoon dried oregano
1/4 teaspoon dried basil
1/4 teaspoon dried dill

Shake all ingredients in tightly covered container. Refrigerate at least 1 hour.

C. MANDARIN SALAD WITH SWEET-SOUR DRESSING

1/4 cup almonds, sliced
1 tablespoon plus 1 teaspoon sugar
1/4 head lettuce, torn into bite-size pieces

1/4 bunch romaine, torn into bite-size pieces
2 medium stalks celery, chopped (about 1 cup)
1 can (11 ounces) mandarin orange segments, drained

1. Cook almonds and sugar over low heat, stirring constantly, until sugar is melted and almonds are coated; cool and break apart.
2. Prepare Sweet-Sour Dressing (below).
3. Place lettuce and Romaine in salad bowl; add celery and onions.
4. Add orange segments. Add Salad Dressing.
5. Toss until all ingredients are evenly coated; add almonds and toss lightly.

Sweet-Sour Dressing

2 tablespoons vegetable oil
1 tablespoon sugar
2 tablespoons cider vinegar

1/2 teaspoon salt
dash of black pepper

Shake all ingredients in tightly covered container; refrigerate.

D. TRICOLOR CABBAGE SLAW

2 cups green cabbage, finely shredded
2 cups red cabbage, finely shredded
1/2 small green pepper, chopped (about 1/4 cup)
1 large carrot, peeled and grated
1/3 cup white vinegar
1 tablespoon vegetable oil

2 tablespoons sugar
1 teaspoon instant onion
1 teaspoon salt
1/2 teaspoon celery seed
1/2 teaspoon dry mustard
1/4 teaspoon pepper

1. Mix all ingredients; cover and refrigerate 3 hours. Just before serving, drain salad.

E. CREAMY CUCUMBER SALAD

1/2 cup plain yogurt
1/2 teaspoon salt
1/4 teaspoon dried dill weed

1/8 teaspoon black pepper
2 medium cucumbers, thinly sliced
1 small onion, thinly sliced and separated into rings

Mix all ingredients. Cover and refrigerate at least 4 hours.

F. TOSSED SALAD WITH PECANS AND STRAWBERRIES AND POPPY SEED DRESSING

4 cups salad greens (combination of leaf lettuce, Romaine, spinach)
1/2 cup pecans, toasted

1 cup fresh strawberries, sliced

Dressing:

1/3 cup cider vinegar
2 tablespoons sugar
1 teaspoon salt
2 tablespoons vegetable oil

1 tablespoon Dijon mustard
1 teaspoon poppy seeds
1/4 teaspoon pepper

1. Wash and dry salad greens.

2.	Prepare dressing and refrigerate until ready to serve. All ingredients are placed in a measuring cup and must be mixed thoroughly.
3.	Toss greens, pecans, and sliced strawberries with dressing. It is not necessary to use all the dressing.
4.	Serve salad immediately.

## III.	MAIN DISH SALADS

### A.	ZIPPY PASTA SALAD (MAIN COURSE)

8 ounces multi-colored pasta spirals
1 tablespoon oil
1 1/2 cups broccoli flowerettes, blanched

1/4 cup red onion, chopped
2 ounces pepperoni, sliced
1 ounce ripe pitted olives, drained and sliced

Dressing

1 tablespoon Dijon-style mustard
1/4 cup red wine vinegar
1 tablespoon sugar
1/2 teaspoon salt
dash of black pepper

1 garlic clove, finely minced
2 tablespoons fresh parsley, finely minced
1/4 cup oil
1/2 cup Parmesan cheese, grated

1.	Cook pasta according to directions; drain and chill in ice water. Drain; add 1 tablespoon oil; refrigerate.
2.	Blanch broccoli; drain and chill in ice water; drain.
3.	Mix broccoli with pasta, red onion, pepperoni, and olives.
4.	In a small bowl, mix mustard, vinegar, sugar, salt, pepper, garlic, and parsley.
5.	Use electric mixer to blend thoroughly, while slowly adding oil.
6.	Add dressing and Parmesan cheese to pasta mixture; mix well. Chill. May be served on lettuce leaf.

### B.	CHEF'S SALAD

1/2 cup 1/4 inch strips meat, cooked (beef, smoked ham, or tongue)
1/2 cup 1/4 inch strips chicken or turkey, cooked
1/2 cup 1/4 inch strips Swiss cheese
1/2 cup green onions (with tops), chopped
1 medium head lettuce, torn into bite-size pieces
1 small bunch Romaine, torn into bite-size pieces

1 medium stalk celery, sliced (about 1/2 cup)
1/2 cup mayonnaise or salad dressing
1/4 cup French Dressing (see below)
2 hard-cooked eggs, sliced
2 tomatoes, cut into wedges
pitted ripe olives

1.	Reserve a few strips of meat, chicken, and cheese. Toss remaining meat, chicken, and cheese, the onions, lettuce, romaine, and celery.
2.	Mix mayonnaise and French Dressing; pour on lettuce and toss. Top with reserved meat, chicken, and cheese strips, the eggs, tomatoes, and olives.

French Dressing

1/4 cup olive oil or vegetable oil or combination
2 tablespoons vinegar
2 tablespoons lemon juice

1/2 teaspoon salt
1/4 teaspoon dry mustard
1/4 teaspoon paprika

don't do

Shake all ingredients in tightly covered container; refrigerate. Shake before serving.

C. TUNA-MACARONI SALAD

1 cup elbow or spiral macaroni, uncooked
1 cup cucumber, chopped
1/2 cup low-fat mayonnaise or salad dressing
1 tablespoon onion, finely chopped
2 tablespoons sweet relish

1 tablespoon lemon juice
1/2 teaspoon salt
1/4 teaspoon black pepper
1 can (9 3/4 ounces) tuna in water, drained
4 cups salad greens, torn into bite-size pieces

1. Cook macaroni as directed on package; drain.
2. Rinse under running cold water; drain.
3. Mix macaroni and remaining ingredients except salad greens.
4. Cover and refrigerate at least 1 hour. Spoon onto salad greens. Garnish with tomato wedges, if desired.

D. CHICKEN SALAD CUPS

Chicken-Almond Salad

2 cups chicken or turkey, cooked, cut-up
1/2 cup celery, chopped
1/2 cup almonds, slivered and toasted
1/3 cup mayonnaise or salad dressing

1 tablespoon lemon juice
1/4 teaspoon salt
1/4 teaspoon black pepper
1 jar (2 ounces) sliced pimentos, drained

1. Mix all ingredients; refrigerate until chilled, at least 1 1/2 hours.

Salad Cups

1/2 cup water
1/4 cup margarine or butter
1/2 cup all-purpose flour

1/2 teaspoon poppy seeds
dash of salt
2 eggs

1. Heat oven to 400°F. Grease 6 medium muffin cups, 2 1/2 × 1 1/4 inches.
2. Heat water and margarine to rolling boil in 2 quart saucepan; stir in flour and salt.
3. Stir vigorously over low heat until mixture forms a ball, about 30 seconds; remove from heat. Cool slightly.
4. Beat in eggs and poppy seeds all at once; continue beating until smooth.
5. Spread 2 rounded tablespoons dough in bottom and up side of each muffin cup. Bake until puffed and dry in center, about 30 minutes. Immediately remove from pan; cool.
6. Just before serving, fill each with about 1/4 cup chicken salad.

IV. DESSERT SALADS

A. WINTER FRUIT SALAD WITH LIME-GINGER DRESSING

2 medium apples, cut into 1/4 inch slices
2 oranges, pared and sliced
1 grapefruit, pared and sliced

2 cups seedless grapes
salad greens

1. Prepare Lime-Ginger Dressing (below).
2. Dip apple slices in dressing.
3. Arrange apples, oranges, grapefruit, and grapes on salad greens.
4. Serve with Lime-Ginger Dressing.

Lime-Ginger Dressing

1/3 cup frozen limeade concentrate, thawed
1/3 cup honey
1 tablespoon vegetable oil

1/2 teaspoon ground ginger or 1 tablespoon of finely chopped crystallized ginger

1.   Beat with hand beater until smooth.

B.   EASY FRUIT SALAD

1 cup seedless grapes
1 can (11 ounces) mandarin orange segments, chilled and drained
1 can (8 1/4 ounces) pineapple chunks in syrup, chilled and drained

1 Red Delicious apple, diced
salad greens
Fruit Salad Yogurt Dressing (below)

1.   Mix grapes, orange segments, pineapple chunks, and apple.
2.   Spoon onto salad greens. Serve with Fruit Salad Yogurt Dressing.

Fruit Salad Yogurt Dressing

2/3 cup plain low-fat or non-fat yogurt
1 tablespoon honey

1 tablespoon orange juice
1/8 teaspoon almond extract

Mix all ingredients together.

QUESTIONS

1.   What criteria should be observed in determining the size of the pieces of food to be used in preparing salads?

2.   When fragile ingredients are used in salads, what precautions should be observed?

3.   What points should be observed in the creation of an attractive salad?

4.   Give directions for retaining or restoring the crispness of vegetables.

5.   How can the browning of fruits, such as apples and bananas, be retarded?

6.   Name, define, and give an example of the four different types of salads.

7.   When should the dressing be added to the salad?

LABORATORY 10

Fats and Emulsions

LABORATORY 10
FATS AND EMULSIONS

Fats contribute flavor and tenderness to food, but also serve as a transfer of heat when used as a medium for cooking. Fat and water are insoluble, but when a third agent (an emulsifier) is used, these two liquids are brought together and an emulsion is formed. This laboratory exercise will look at different types of fats, their stability, and the role that fat plays in transferring heat during preparation. The difference between a temporary and a permanent emulsion will also be demonstrated.

VOCABULARY

acrolein	free fatty acid	margarine	polyunsaturated fatty acid
antioxidant	glycerol	monounsaturated fatty acid	rancidity
butter	hydrogenated	oxidation	smoke point
dispersing medium	hydrolytic rancidity	permanent emulsion	temporary emulsion
double bond	immiscible	plastic	triglyceride
emulsifier	lard	phospholipid	winterize
fatty acid			

OBJECTIVES

1.   To show the effect of frying temperature on the quality of the cooked product.
2.   To evaluate various fats according to color, flavor, and aroma.
3.   To be familiar with the rancid quality of a fat or oil.
4.   To emphasize different emulsions and the effect of an emulsifying agent on the formation and stability of the emulsion formed.

PRINCIPLES

1.   Fats can be long or short chained and saturated or unsaturated.
2.   The melting point of a fat is determined by:
     a.   the length of the chain.
     b.   the degree of saturation.
3.   Fats that are used for frying should have a high melting point.
4.   The temperature used for frying is important and will affect the quality of the cooked food.
     a.   Too low a frying temperature will cause absorption of fat.
     b.   Too high a frying temperature will cause burning and undercooking of the product.
5.   During frying, fats come off the triglyceride molecule in the form of free fatty acids. Glycerol is then broken down to acrolein which is irritating to the nose and eyes.
6.   Fats can go rancid in two ways:
     a.   hydrolytic rancidity which is caused by enzymatic action.
     b.   oxidative rancidity which is caused by exposure of the fat to oxygen, light, and metals.
7.   Antioxidants are used in fats and oils to prevent rancidity. Typical examples are: butylated hydroxyanisole (BHA), butylated hydroxytoluene (BHT), tertiary butyl hydroquinone (TBHQ), and propyl gallate.
8.   Fat and water are immiscible and when they come together they form a temporary emulsion. With the aid of an emulsifier a permanent emulsion is formed.
9.   Mayonnaise is an example of a permanent emulsion. French dressing is an example of a temporary emulsion.

CAUTION
Fats and oils can be heated to very high temperatures and are easily ignited when hot. Be careful not to burn yourself or spill oil on a hot burner. In case of fire, smother the fire with a lid or baking soda. DO NOT put water on an oil fire. Place the deep-fat frying pan with the handle away from you and not near the edge of the counter to avoid spills and possible burns.

I. TO SHOW THE EFFECTS OF FRYING TEMPERATURE ON FAT ABSORPTION DURING DEEP FAT FRYING

A. DOUGHNUT HOLES

2 1/4 cups all-purpose flour
2 teaspoons baking powder
1/2 teaspoon salt
dash of nutmeg
1/8 teaspoon cinnamon

1/2 cup sugar
1 tablespoon vegetable oil
1/2 cup milk
1 egg
4 cups vegetable oil for deep fat frying

1. Place fat for frying in a pan 5-6 inches deep with a diameter 6-7 inches. There should be 2-3 inches of melted fat in the pan. Do not use less than 2 inches or more than 3 inches of fat. Hold over low heat while preparing the dough-nut batter.
2. Sift together all dry ingredients into large size bowl.
3. In small size bowl blend together the egg, milk, and vegetable oil. Use a rotary beater for blending. The oil must thoroughly blend with the egg yolk and milk as the liquid mixture is added to the dry ingredients.
4. Add liquid ingredients to dry ingredients and stir 50 strokes. Scrape down sides of bowl and clean spoon with rubber spatula midway in the stirring period.
5. Place dough on lightly floured sheet of waxed paper.
6. Roll dough between two 1/2 inch pastry guides. Cut with doughnut hole cutter.
7. Weigh 2 doughnut holes and record weight: _____. Fry at 325°F. Drain and reweigh; record weight: _____.
8. Cook the remaining doughnut holes (except for 2) for approximately 3 minutes at 365°F. It will be necessary to turn to get even browning during frying.
9. Use a slotted spoon to remove the cooked doughnut holes from the fat. Place doughnut holes on several layers of paper toweling to drain off excess fat.
10. Weigh 2 doughnut holes cooked at 365°F and record weight: _____.
11. Raise temperature to 390°F and cook the 2 remaining doughnut holes.
12. Weigh the 2 doughnut holes and record weight: _____.
13. Calculate % fat absorption using the following formula:

$$\frac{\text{cooked weight} - \text{precooked weight}}{\text{precooked weight}} \times 100$$

14. For evaluation **do not** roll doughnut holes in sugar. Doughnut holes not used for evaluation may be rolled in sugar.
15. Evaluation: Cut doughnut holes in half. Examine for penetration of oil used for frying. It will appear as a ring inside the doughnut hole.

TABLE FOR EVALUATION OF DOUGHNUT HOLES				
Frying Temperature	Original Weight (gm)	Fry Time (min)	Drained Weight (gm)	Penetration of Fat
325°F				
365°F				
390°F				

QUESTIONS

1. State and account for the effects of frying temperature on fat absorption.

2. a. How was the color of the frying oil at the beginning and at the end of the frying period?

   b. What caused the color change?

3. Describe the desirable characteristics of fried foods.

4. What is the smoke point of a fat and what factors affect it?

5. a. What is the irritating ingredient in the smoke from fat?

   b. What is its source?

6. What are the structural differences between a saturated fatty acid and an unsaturated fatty acid?

II. TO EVALUATE FATS ACCORDING TO COLOR, FLAVOR, AND AROMA AND TO BE ABLE TO DETECT RANCIDITY IN A FAT

A. IDENTIFICATION OF FATS AND OILS

A series of fats and oils will be displayed for evaluation of aroma, color, and flavor. Both fresh and rancid varieties will be presented for identification. List the fats in the table provided for evaluation.

TABLE FOR EVALUATION OF FATS AND OILS				
Type of Fat	Source	Color	Odor	Flavor

QUESTIONS

1. What causes a fat to become rancid?

2. What is the difference between butter and margarine?

3. What is meant by a refined oil?

4. What steps must be taken to prevent rancidity in a fat?

5. a. What is an antioxidant and identify those that are used in fats and oils?

   b. What natural antioxidant is found in oil?

6. What is a synergist and describe its action in a fat or oil?

7. Name the types of lard and how they are processed.

III. **TO BECOME FAMILIAR WITH VARIOUS EMULSIONS AND THE EFFECT THAT THE EMULSIFIER HAS ON STABILIZING THE EMULSION**

 A. **FRENCH DRESSING (TEMPORARY EMULSION)**

1 teaspoon sugar	dash of cayenne pepper
1/2 teaspoon salt	2 tablespoons lemon juice
1/2 teaspoon dry mustard	2 tablespoons vinegar
1/2 teaspoon paprika	1/2 cup salad oil

1. Place all ingredients in a covered jar.
2. Shake well before using.

B. MAYONNAISE (PERMANENT EMULSION)

2 egg yolks
1/2 teaspoon salt
1/8 teaspoon paprika
1/4 teaspoon dry mustard

dash of cayenne pepper
1 tablespoon vinegar
1 tablespoon lemon juice
1 cup salad oil

1. Place egg yolks in a **small**, deep bowl (1 quart). Add salt, paprika, mustard, and cayenne pepper and blend with egg.
2. Add vinegar and mix well.
3. Add salad oil, a few droplets at a time, beating with hand mixer until 1/2 cup has been added.
4. Add lemon juice; beat until incorporated.
5. Add salad oil, 1 tablespoon at a time, beating well after each addition.

NOTE: "Due to the risk of raw eggs containing *Salmonella,* mayonnaise should not be tasted."

C. BLENDER MAYONNAISE (PERMANENT EMULSION)

1 egg
1/2 teaspoon dry mustard
1/2 teaspoon sugar

1/2 teaspoon salt
2 tablespoons vinegar (white or cider)
1 cup salad oil

1. Put egg, seasonings, vinegar, and 1/4 cup of oil into blender container.
2. Cover and process at BLEND.
3. Immediately remove feeder cap and pour in the remaining oil in a steady stream. (If necessary, STOP BLENDER, use rubber spatula to keep mixture around processing blades. Cover and continue to process.)
4. Store covered in the refrigerator up to 1 week.

Variation: For low cholesterol mayonnaise, use 2 egg whites instead of 1 whole egg. Proceed as above.

NOTE: "Due to the risk of raw eggs containing *Salmonella,* mayonnaise should not be tasted."

D. COOKED DRESSING (Permanent Emulsion)

2 tablespoons sugar
1 teaspoon salt
2 tablespoons flour
1 teaspoon dry mustard
few grains cayenne pepper

2 egg yolks, slightly beaten
3/4 cup milk
1/4 cup mild vinegar
1 tablespoon butter or margarine

1. Mix sugar, salt, flour, mustard, and cayenne pepper.
2. Add egg yolks and milk and blend.
3. Cook in double boiler until thick, stirring continuously for 10-12 minutes.
4. Remove from heat. Add butter and vinegar.

TABLE FOR EVALUATION OF EMULSIONS				
Product	Type of Emulsion	Stability	Appearance	Flavor
French Dressing				
Mayonnaise				
Blender Mayonnaise				
Cooked Dressing				

QUESTIONS

1.   What are the essential ingredients in:

   a.   French dressing?

   b.   mayonnaise?

   c.   cooked dressing?

2.   What is a permanent emulsion? Give an example.

3.   What is a temporary emulsion? Give an example.

4.   What is the function of dry mustard, paprika, and cayenne pepper in French dressing?

5.   Why does mayonnaise thicken?

6.   a.   What may cause the emulsion in mayonnaise to break?

   b.   How can the emulsion be reformed?

7.   Oil and vinegar dressings require an oil that remains liquid when refrigerated. What kind of oil should be used?

LABORATORY 11

Gelatin

LABORATORY 11
GELATIN

Gelatin is used primarily in food preparation to thicken and form a gel. There are two types of gelatin: coarse grind ("Knox" unflavored) and fine grind ("Jello"). These two types are dissolved differently, but the final results are achieved in a gel (liquid trapped in a solid). The purpose of this laboratory exercise is to introduce the student to the proper handling techniques for gelatin in food preparation; and how it can be utilized and manipulated in a variety of products.

VOCABULARY

bromelin	foam	sol
bavarian cream	gel	Spanish cream
chiffon	gelatin	sponge
collagen		

OBJECTIVES

1. To compare products made with unflavored gelatin and the available commercial mix.
2. To understand how to dissolve and melt the gelatin for product making.
3. To become familiar with the setting mechanism of gelatin.
4. To identify uses of gelatin in foams, molded salads, and desserts.

PRINCIPLES

1. Gelatin is derived from bones, hides, and connective tissues (collagen) of animals.
2. There are two marketed forms of gelatin: unflavored gelatin granules and flavored, sweetened granular gelatin.
3. The unflavored gelatin has coarse granules, whereby, the flavored gelatin is pulverized and finer granules are present.
4. When gelatin is dissolved in water, the water molecules bond to the protein and the protein molecules swell slightly. Heating of the gelatin and the water forms a dispersion known as a sol (solid in a liquid).
5. Upon cooling, the hydrogen bonds come together, trap the water, and a gel is formed (liquid in a solid).
6. Slow cooling of a sol produces a stronger gel than rapid cooling, permitting a more ordered formation of the bonds between the protein chains.
7. Too much acid can weaken the gel.
8. Proteolytic enzymes will prevent bond formation in the gelatin. Fresh pineapple contains bromelin and cannot be added to a gelatin mold.
9. When adding solid ingredients such as chopped meat, vegetables, fruits, and nuts to a gelatin mixture, the gelatin sol must be partially set, thus preventing floatation.
10. When creating gelatin foams, the sol must be partially set, or egg white consistency in nature, before beating.
11. When the mold is completely gelled, dip it into a container of warm water for a few seconds then invert it onto the serving dish (*FIG. 1*).
12. Gelatin is deficient in the essential amino acid tryptophan and, therefore, cannot support the growth of young animals.

FIG. 1. To unmold gelatin, quickly dip the mold into warm water (A) to loosen the gelatin. Insert a spatula or knife blade to one side to let air in (B). Place an inverted plate over the mold (C) and invert the mold and plate together (D).

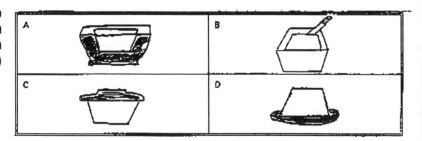

TO COMPARE PRODUCTS MADE WITH UNFLAVORED GELATIN AND THE AVAILABLE COMMERCIAL MIX

1. Follow instructions on a 3 ounce package of commercial gelatin dessert (orange flavor). Pour 1/2 of the dissolved mixture into a mold and chill. For the remainder, follow instructions for Orange Whip (steps 2-5).
2. Prepare homemade orange jelly.
3. Record the time for each to set.
4. Rank the gels for stiffness, flavor, and clarity.

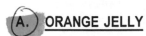 **ORANGE JELLY**

1 1/2 teaspoons unflavored gelatin	2 tablespoons lemon juice
2 tablespoons cold water	6 tablespoons orange juice
1/3 cup hot water	1/4 cup sugar

1. Hydrate gelatin in cold water.
2. Add hot water and stir to disperse gelatin.
3. Add sugar and dissolve. Cool. Add fruit juices.
4. Pour into container or molds and place in refrigerator to set.

B. ORANGE WHIP

1. Use the same ingredients as in A and combine for orange jelly.
2. Place in refrigerator to chill.
3. When the gelatin is the consistency of thick egg white, whip until the foam holds its shape.
4. Pour into a container or mold and return to refrigerator to set.
5. Observe the amount of volume which increased due to beating.

TABLE FOR EVALUATION OF ORANGE GELATIN				
Type	Time to Set	Stiffness	Flavor	Clarity
Commercial				
Commercial-Whip				
Orange Jelly				
Orange Whip				

QUESTIONS

1. Approximately how much gelatin is needed to gel 2 cups of liquid?

2. What effect does acid have upon a gelatin gel?

3. a. List the ways to speed the gelling of gelatin mixtures.

97

b.   Is this advantageous to the mixture?

4.   Describe briefly the methods recommended for dispersing the two market forms of gelatin.

II. TO IDENTIFY AND TO BECOME FAMILIAR WITH THE DIFFERENT USES OF GELATIN

A. CARROT-PINEAPPLE SALAD

6 ounce can frozen orange juice concentrate, thawed
2/3 cup water
1 package (3 ounces) orange-flavor gelatin
2/3 cup lemon-lime flavored carbonated beverage, chilled

1/8 teaspoon salt
1 can (8 1/4 ounces) crushed pineapple in syrup
1 cup carrot (about 1 medium), shredded

1.   In large saucepan, heat orange juice concentrate and water to boiling; stir in gelatin until dissolved.
2.   Slowly add carbonated beverage; add salt.
3.   Refrigerate until thickened but not set.
4.   Fold in crushed pineapple and shredded carrots.
5.   Pour into 4 cup mold.
6.   Refrigerate until firm.
7.   Unmold onto lettuce lined serving plate.

B. SPANISH CREAM

1 tablespoon gelatin
1/4 cup cold milk
1 1/3 cups scalded milk
2 eggs, separated

1/3 cup sugar
1/8 teaspoon salt
1 teaspoon vanilla extract

1.   Place cold milk in a custard cup; add the gelatin; let stand while making a stirred custard from the scalded milk, salt, 2 tablespoons of the sugar, and the egg yolks. Cook this custard mixture over warm not boiling water, until the mixture "coats" the spoon.
2.   Add the hydrated gelatin to the warm custard. Stir until the gelatin is dissolved. Add the vanilla; chill.
3.   Beat the egg whites until they form soft peaks. Gradually add remaining sugar with some beating. Peaks should remain slightly soft.
4.   Add the gelatin mixture and fold until just blended. Place in gelatin mold. Chill until firm.
5.   Serve with whipped cream and/or frozen raspberries.

C. PINEAPPLE-COCONUT BAVARIAN CREAM

2 teaspoons gelatin
1/4 cup cold water
1/4 cup sugar
1/2 cup sweetened coconut, divided

1 cup crushed pineapple* with syrup
1 tablespoon lemon juice
3/4 cup whipping cream

1.   Put 1/4 cup cold water in a 2 quart bowl. Add the gelatin. Let stand.
2.   Drain syrup from pineapple; add enough water to make 1/2 cup liquid; bring to a boil.
3.   Add the boiling liquid to gelatin; stir until gelatin is dissolved.
*Fresh or frozen pineapple **cannot** be used in gelatin products.

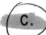

4. Add the sugar and stir until dissolved; add lemon juice.
5. Chill in ice bath until it is the consistency of raw egg white. Beat with electric mixer until light and foamy (soft peak stage). (Wash the beaters before going to step 6.)
6. Whip the whipping cream (be careful and do not make butter); fold the whipped cream, 1/4 cup coconut, and pineapple into the whipped gelatin. Do not overfold! Pile into mold; chill.
7. Toast remaining coconut in a 350°F oven for 5-6 minutes. Unmold the bavarian and sprinkle with toasted coconut.

D. STRAWBERRY CHIFFON

1 tablespoon gelatin	1 pound frozen strawberries
1/4 cup cold water	1 egg white
1/4 cup sugar*	3/4 cup whipping cream
1 tablespoon lemon juice	

1. Put water in upper part of double boiler. Add gelatin; let stand 5 minutes.
2. Dissolve gelatin over boiling water. Add sugar, berries, and lemon juice and cook until all ingredients are heated.
3. Remove from heat. Chill mixture until it mounds from a spoon. Beat mixture until light and foamy with electric mixer (soft peak stage). (Wash beaters before going to step 4.)
4. Beat egg white to soft peak stage. Fold into gelatin mixture. (Wash beaters from going to step 5.)
5. Beat whipping cream into a foam; fold into gelatin mixture. Pile into mold; chill until firm.
*Increase sugar to 1/2 cup if fresh or unsweetened berries are used.

E. LIME BAVARIAN

2/3 cup evaporated milk	2 tablespoons lime juice
1 1/2 ounces lime gelatin (1/2 of a 3 ounce package)	1 tablespoon lemon juice
2 tablespoons water	1 teaspoon lime rind, grated
1 teaspoon plain gelatin	1 1/2 cups chocolate wafer crumbs
3/4 cup boiling water	1/3 cup margarine
1/2 cup sugar	1 ounce semisweet chocolate, grated

1. Chill the evaporated milk in a 9 inch glass pie pan in the freezer until ice crystals are formed on the insides of the pan (30 minutes).
2. Place chocolate wafer cookies on bread board; crush to fine crumbs with rolling pin. Melt margarine; add wafer crumbs; blend; press evenly into 9 inch pie dish; chill.
3. In a custard cup add 2 tablespoons water and 1 teaspoon plain gelatin. Allow to soften for 5 minutes.
4. In a 2 quart bowl, blend lime gelatin, and sugar; add boiling water and unflavored gelatin (step 3); stir until gelatins and sugar are dissolved; add lime and lemon juices.
5. Chill mixture in a pan of chipped ice until gelatin is the consistency of a raw egg white.
6. Remove bowl from ice; use an electric mixer to beat to soft peak stage. Blend in the lime rind with the electric mixer. (Wash beaters before going to step 7.)
7. Quickly beat the evaporated milk until it forms soft peaks.
8. Add the beaten milk to the beaten gelatin, beating with the hand mixer.
9. Pour and/or spoon the blended mixture over the chocolate crumbs.
10. Sprinkle shredded chocolate over the top. Chill.

I. **WHITE COCONUT CHIFFON**

1 tablespoon unflavored gelatin
1/4 cup all-purpose flour
1/2 teaspoon salt
1/2 cup sugar
1 3/4 cups 1 1/2% milk
1 teaspoon vanilla

1/4 teaspoon almond extract
4 egg whites
1/2 cup sugar
1/4 teaspoon cream of tartar
1/2 cup flaked sweetened coconut

1. In a 2 quart saucepan, blend together unflavored gelatin, flour, 1/2 cup sugar, and salt.
2. Slowly add milk and blend making sure no lumps are present.
3. Cook over medium heat, stirring constantly. Bring to a boil and remove from heat.
4. Add vanilla and almond extracts. Cool until mixture mounds slightly when dropped from a spoon.
5. Beat egg whites until foamy; add cream of tartar. Beat until soft peaks form. Add remaining sugar (1/2 cup), 1 tablespoon at a time. Beat until sugar is dissolved and egg whites form a stiff peak.
6. Fold cooled mixture into meringue; fold in coconut.
7. Pour mixture into a baked crust or individual dessert dishes. Refrigerate until set: 4 hours.

Variation: For a special treat divide coconut and dye it with various food colors (e.g., red and blue against the white background).

QUESTIONS

1. Would you advise serving a tart molded gelatin salad on a hot day? Why?

2. What is the difference between a bavarian and a chiffon?

3. Give an example of how a gelatin can be used for different parts of a meal.

4. Since your fingernails are composed mainly of collagen, gelatin should be consumed to strengthen nails. True or False? Explain.

LABORATORY 12

Egg Cookery

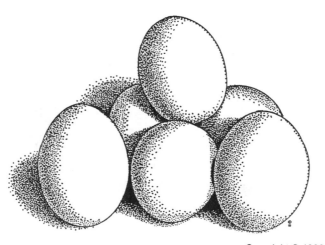

Copyright © 1993 Metro ImageBase, Inc.

LABORATORY 12
EGG COOKERY

Eggs serve important functional roles in food preparation: foaming; coagulation, gelling; emulsification, binding, leavening; flavor; color; and nutritive value. The purpose of this laboratory exercise is to introduce the student to the different preparation techniques that are utilized with eggs.

VOCABULARY

candling	curdling	stirred custard
chalaza	denature	syneresis
coagulate	ferrous sulfide	vitelline membrane

OBJECTIVES

1. To illustrate factors which affect the quality of cooked eggs.
2. To understand how heat affects gelation of egg proteins.
3. To observe the use of egg white foams in food preparation.
4. To become familiar with the different uses of eggs in food preparation.

PRINCIPLES

1. The basic parts of the egg are the shell, the white, and the yolk.
2. The fragile membrane, the **vitelline membrane**, covers the yolk, separating it from the white. Attached to opposite sides of the yolk are threads of thick white called **chalazae**, that help keep the yolk centered in the white inside the egg (*FIG.1*).

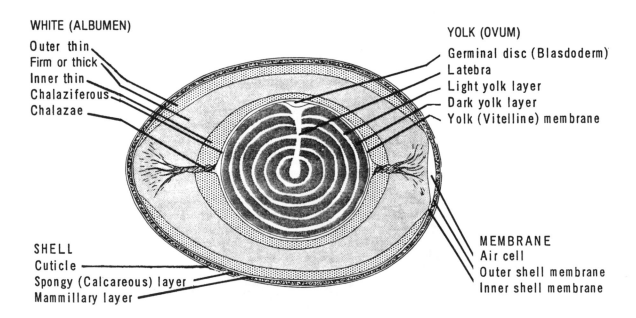

FIG1. The parts of an egg.

3. The shell of the egg is porous and allows gases and moisture to pass in and out.
4. Eggs are graded from highest to lowest quality: U.S. Grade AA, U.S. Grade A, and U.S. Grade B.

5. Several changes occur in eggs over time:
   a. size of air cell increases.
   b. carbon dioxide is lost; the egg becomes more alkaline.
   c. increased alkalinity causes thinning of the white.
   d. yolk enlarges and becomes flatter due to the entrance of water from the white.
   e. flavor and aroma deterioration.
6. Eggs serve several functions in food preparation:
   a. thickening agent in sauces and custards.
   b. gelling agent in baked custard.
   c. structural ingredient in baked products.
   d. leavening agent, incorporating air with egg foams.
   e. source of water in cookie doughs and sponge cakes.
   f. emulsifier in mayonnaise, hollandaise, cakes, and cream puffs.
   g. binding agent in meat loaves, croquettes, for breading on meats, and casseroles.
   h. "eggs" prepared in a variety of ways.
   i. ingredient in many dishes where they serve no particular function other than to provide nutrition, flavor, texture, or color.
7. Heat affects the protein of an egg.
8. Gelation and coagulation are terms used to describe the effect of heat on eggs. **Gelation** is the formation of a gel structure by heat, as in baked custards. **Coagulation** is the change from the liquid to solid state with no particular structure (it occurs in stirred custard and in fried or boiled eggs).
9. Eggs are a good source of complete protein, but also an excellent supplier of vitamin A, iron, riboflavin, and other vitamins and minerals. Eggs are also a rich source of cholesterol.
10. When whipped, raw egg white traps air pulled in by the beaters into bubbles surrounded by a film of protein molecules. Egg whites retain more air when beaten at room temperature.

I. TO OBSERVE THE EFFECT OF AGING ON THE RAW EGG

1. Use an egg candler to observe the shell and inside of an old egg and a fresh egg.
2. Break the eggs and observe on a flat plate, 6-7 inches in diameter.
3. Record your observations.

TABLE FOR EVALUATION OF RAW EGGS		
Characteristic	Old	New
Size of Air Sac		
Amount of Thick White		
Amount of Thin White		
Height of Yolk		

QUESTIONS

1. Why was there an increase in the thinning of the egg white?

2. Why did the yolk get flatter?

3. How would you use these eggs for preparation?

II. TO BECOME FAMILIAR WITH VARIOUS METHODS TO COOK EGGS

A. POACHED EGGS

1. Fill pan with enough water to cover the egg.
2. Heat to simmering.
3. Carefully break a fresh egg and an old egg into separate custard cups. Slip one egg into the hot water.
4. Cover pan and keep water hot but below simmering. Cook until the white is firm and the yolk is of desired consistency (3-5 minutes).
5. Remove egg with a perforated turner or slotted spoon.
6. Repeat process with other egg.

Variation: Affect of Vortex Action and Acid on Poached Egg

1. Break an egg into custard cup.
2. Bring water to simmering. Stir water rapidly and quickly slip egg into the vortex.
3. Add lemon juice to water (2 teaspoons to 1 quart water). This tends to hasten the coagulation of the egg.

TABLE FOR EVALUATION OF POACHED EGGS		
Egg	Appearance of White	Appearance of Yolk
Old Egg		
Fresh Egg		
Fresh Egg: Vortex + Lemon Juice		

QUESTIONS

1. What effect did the acid have on the egg?

2. Compare the old egg vs. the fresh egg as to appearance.

B. COOKED EGG IN THE SHELL (Hard Cooked)

1. Place 2 eggs in a pan and cover with water.
2. Heat the water to boiling in a deep covered saucepan.
3. Boil for :
   a. 10 minutes and remove egg and cool rapidly under cold running water.
   b. Continue cooking the other egg for another 10 minutes (total cooking time: 20 minutes); remove from water, but allow it to cool to room temperature.

TABLE FOR EVALUATION OF HARD BOILED EGGS				
Treatment	Presence of Sulfur Ring	Texture of Yolk	Texture of White	Odor
10 minutes and cooled				
20 minutes and no cooling				

104

QUESTION

1.   Why does the sulfur ring appear? What can be done to avoid it?

C.   FRIED EGG

Variation 1: Fat Only

1.   Heat 1 tablespoon butter or margarine in an 8 inch skillet over moderate heat.
2.   Break egg into heated skillet.
3.   Reduce heat slightly and cook, basting with fat until desired firmness.

Variation 2: Fat and Water

1.   Heat 2 teaspoons butter or margarine in an 8 inch skillet over moderate heat.
2.   Break egg into heated skillet.
3.   Add 2 tablespoons water and cover (the steam helps to form a coating over the yolk).
4.   Reduce heat and cook at low temperature until white has coagulated.

TABLE FOR EVALUATION OF FRIED EGGS				
Variation	Appearance of Yolk	Texture of Yolk	Texture of White	Flavor
1				
2				

D.   SCRAMBLED EGGS

2 eggs   few grains of salt
2 tablespoons milk or cream   1 teaspoon fat

1.   Beat eggs, milk, and seasonings together.
2.   Melt fat in pan.
3.   Add egg mixture. Stir when egg has coagulated, lifting watery part. Stir gently until all mass has coagulated.

E.   SCRAMBLED EGGS - MICROWAVE OVEN METHOD

2 eggs   1/8 teaspoon salt
2 tablespoons milk   1 teaspoon butter or margarine

1.   Place butter or margarine into a 2 cup microwave cooking container. Microwave at high for 15 seconds or until fat is melted.
2.   In a small size bowl combine eggs, milk, and salt. Beat with a rotary beater until yolks and whites are thoroughly blended, but not foamy. Pour into melted fat.
3.   Microwave at high for 30 seconds; stir. Microwave for another 30 seconds at high power; stir.
4.   Microwave for another 30 seconds at high; at this point the eggs will appear moist and slightly creamy; they are servable as the eggs will continue to cook for a short time. However, the eggs can be cooked to a greater degree of doneness by heating at 5 second intervals. Care must be used to avoid overcooking.

F.   SCRAMBLED "EGG BEATERS" (COMMERCIAL EGG SUBSTITUTE)

1/2 cup egg beaters, thawed   1 teaspoon margarine

1. Melt margarine in heavy frying pan over medium high heat.
2. When margarine is hot (not smoking) pour in egg beaters. **Do not stir**.
3. When egg beaters begin to become firm around edges, push set portion to center of pan, allowing uncooked portion to flow to edges of pan. **DO NOT STIR**. Turn over to cook to desired doneness. Season as desired.

TABLE FOR EVALUATION OF SCRAMBLED EGGS			
Type	Moistness	Texture	Color
Conventional			
Microwaved			
Egg Beaters			

CHARACTERISTICS OF HIGH QUALITY SCRAMBLED EGGS

Appearance: Even masses appear slightly moist and creamy; usually egg masses are large.
Consistency: Even consistency throughout; all liquid is held by coagulated protein.
Tenderness: Egg masses are tender and have little resistance when cut or chewed.
Flavor: Mild egg flavor; fat used will enhance (example: butter, bacon).

G. FRENCH OMELET (PLAIN OMELET)

1. Use recipe for scrambled eggs.
2. Lift cooked eggs with spatula and let uncooked liquid run to bottom of skillet. Keep omelet uniformly thick.
3. Roll and serve.

H. PUFFY OMELET

4 eggs, separated   1/4 teaspoon cream of tartar
1/4 cup water   1 tablespoon margarine
1/4 teaspoon salt

1. Beat egg yolks until thick and lemon colored, about 5 minutes.
2. Add water, salt, and cream of tartar to whites; beat until stiff but not dry or just until whites no longer slip when bowl is tilted.
3. Fold yolks into whites.
4. On medium-high heat, heat margarine in 10 inch omelet pan or skillet with ovenproof handle until just hot enough to sizzle a drop of water.
5. Pour in omelet mixture; level surface gently. Reduce heat to medium. Cook slowly until puffy and lightly browned on bottom, about 5 minutes.
6. Lift omelet at edge to judge color. Bake in preheated 350°F oven 10-12 minutes or until knife inserted halfway between center and outside edge comes out clean.

TABLE FOR EVALUATION OF OMELETS			
Omelet	Texture	Appearance	Flavor
Plain Omelet (French Omelet)			
Puffy Omelet			

QUESTIONS

1. Discuss the effect of cooking method on the flavor and caloric content of fried eggs.

2. Distinguish between scrambled eggs, French omelet, and puffy omelet.

3. What was the difference between the scrambled eggs and Egg Beaters?

4. What precautions should be taken when microwaving scrambled eggs?

III. TO UNDERSTAND HOW HEAT AFFECTS GELATION OF EGG PROTEINS

A. BAKED CUSTARD

2 eggs, slightly beaten	1 1/2 cups very warm milk
2 1/2 tablespoons sugar	1/2 teaspoon vanilla
dash salt	nutmeg, as desired

1. Preheat oven to 350°F.
2. Combine eggs, sugar, and salt.
3. Stir in the milk gradually.
4. Add vanilla.
5. Pour mixture evenly into 3 custard cups.
6. Sprinkle with nutmeg.
7. Place cups in square pan, 8 × 8 × 2 inches, on oven rack. Pour very hot water into pan to within 1/2 inch of tops of cups.
8. Bake about 45 minutes, or until custard is set.

NOTE: Baked custard is done when the tip of a table knife inserted in the center comes out clean.

B. STIRRED CUSTARD WITH FLOATING ISLAND

1 1/2 cups milk	1/4 cup sugar
2 egg yolks	1/2 teaspoon vanilla extract
1 whole egg	

1. Blend together milk, egg, yolks, and sugar. **Do not beat because the mixture becomes foamy.**
2. Put custard mixture into the upper part of a double boiler. **Water in the lower part should be simmering.**
3. Stir custard constantly with a wooden spoon.
4. Cook until custard coats a metal spoon. ⟵ thickley
5. Cool custard immediately by removing from pot. Add vanilla.

Meringue (Floating Island)

2 egg whites	1/4 teaspoon vanilla extract
1/4 cup sugar	

1. Preheat oven to 350°F.
2. Place egg whites into smallest size bowl. Add vanilla. Beat with mixer until the whites form soft peaks.
3. Add the sugar gradually, beating only enough after each addition to blend sugar with foam. At the end of the beating period the egg whites should form fairly stiff peaks which slightly bend over at the tips.
4. Place 1/2 inch hot water in a 9 × 13 × 2 inch pan.

5. Place the meringue on the hot water using a teaspoon to form 10 "islands".
6. Bake in a 350°F oven until meringue is set and the tips are golden brown - approximately 20 minutes.
7. Use slotted pancake turner to remove "islands" from the hot water onto a plate for cooling.
8. Place cooled "islands" on cooled stirred custard before serving.

C. LOW-FAT STIRRED CUSTARD

2 cups skim evaporated milk   2 eggs, thoroughly beaten
3 tablespoons light brown sugar   1 teaspoon vanilla extract

1. Heat water in the bottom part of a double boiler.
2. To the top part add milk and brown sugar.
3. Place over boiling water and scald.
4. Lower temperature of water to simmering.
5. Add a small amount of scalded milk to beaten eggs; stir and mix thoroughly; return to milk.
6. Place double boiler back on top of simmering water and continue cooking, stirring constantly until mixture coats a spoon.
7. Remove from heat and add vanilla extract; pour into bowl to cool.

Suggestions: Excellent over fresh fruit: strawberries, raspberries.

TABLE FOR EVALUATION OF CUSTARDS				
Type	Firmness of Gel	Syneresis	Flavor	Color
Baked				
Stirred				
Stirred/Floating Island				
Stirred - Low-Fat				

QUESTIONS

1. What is a custard?

   How do baked and stirred custards differ?

2. List desirable characteristics of stirred and baked custards.

3. Describe the mechanism of gelation in a baked custard.

4. What is the difference in the gel formation from gelatin and gel formation in custards?

5.   Why must both time and temperature be controlled in cooking custard mixtures?

6.   Describe how to determine when baked and stirred custards are done.

IV.   TO OBSERVE THE USE OF EGG WHITE FOAMS IN FOOD PREPARATION

A.)   CHEESE SOUFFLE

2 tablespoons all-purpose flour	3/4 cup cheddar cheese, shredded
1/4 teaspoon salt	few grains of cayenne pepper
2/3 cup milk	2 egg yolks
1 tablespoon margarine	3 egg whites

1.   Preheat oven to 350°F. Separate eggs.
2.   Blend flour, salt, and cayenne pepper together in a saucepan. Add the cold milk gradually and stir until the flour is evenly dispersed.
3.   Place on heat and bring to a boil with constant stirring. Boil 1 minute until the sauce is thick. Remove from heat.
4.   Add the margarine and shredded cheese to the hot sauce. Stir until cheese has melted.
5.   Add the unbeaten yolks to the sauce; stir until eggs are blended.
6.   Beat egg whites until they form stiff peaks.
7.   Add the sauce mixture to the egg whites; fold with a rubber spatula until all ingredients are blended. Fold lightly; do not overblend.
8.   Lightly butter the bottom of a small size (1 quart) souffle dish. Pour in souffle mixture. Set the dish in a pan of warm water - **water should be the same depth as the amount of souffle in its baking dish**.
9.   Place in oven and bake until a knife inserted in the center comes out clean, about 50 minutes. Serve immediately.

B.)   CHOCOLATE SOUFFLE ROLL

1 package (6 ounces) semisweet chocolate morsels	2 teaspoons cocoa
2 tablespoons black coffee	5 tablespoons confectioner's sugar
6 eggs, separated	1 cup whipping cream
1/2 cup sugar	1 teaspoon vanilla extract
1 teaspoon vanilla extract	

1.   Grease bottom and sides of a 15 × 10 × 1 inch jellyroll pan with vegetable oil; line with waxed paper (have waxed paper overhang at both ends), and grease waxed paper with oil. Set aside.
2.   Place chocolate morsels and black coffee in top of a double boiler; bring water to a boil. Reduce heat to low; stirring occasionally, until chocolate melts.
3.   Beat egg yolks in a large bowl at high speed of an electric mixer until foamy. Gradually add sugar, beating until mixture is thick and lemon colored (the mixture will look much like cake batter). Stir in 1 teaspoon vanilla extract.
4.   Gradually stir in melted chocolate; make sure chocolate is well distributed and there are no yellow streaks.
5.   Beat egg whites until stiff peaks are formed (remember overbeating will cause brittle and dry egg white foam).
6.   Stir a small amount of egg white foam into chocolate mixture. This "lightens" the mixture and will prevent deflation of the foam.
7.   Fold remainder of egg whites into chocolate mixture.
8.   Pour chocolate mixture into prepared pan, spreading evenly. Bake at 350°F for 15-18 minutes in middle of oven; do not overbake.
9.   Remove from oven and immediately cover top with a damp cloth towel; place on a wire rack, and let cool 1 hour. Carefully remove towel. Loosen edges with a metal spatula.

10. Place 2 lengths of wax paper (longer than jellyroll pan) on a smooth slightly damp surface. Tape the waxed paper together (overlap the two pieces then tape). Sprinkle with a combination of 2 teaspoons cocoa and 3 tablespoons of confectioner's sugar.
11. Quickly invert jellyroll pan on waxed paper with long side nearest you; remove pan, and carefully peel paper from chocolate roll.
12. Beat heavy cream with 2 tablespoons of confectioner's sugar and 1 teaspoon vanilla; beat until stiff peaks are formed.
13. Spoon whipped cream over chocolate roll, spreading it so that there is more on the side facing you (mixture will spread out as you roll); leave a 1-inch margin on all sides.
14. Starting at long side, carefully roll jellyroll fashion; use the waxed paper to help support the souffle as you roll. Secure waxed paper around souffle; smooth and shape it with your hands.
15. Carefully slide roll onto a large baking sheet, seam side down; store in refrigerator until serving time.
16. Before serving, sift additional confectioner's sugar over.

Variation: In place of the vanilla whipped cream, substitute chocolate whipped cream.

Chocolate Whipped Cream

1 cup heavy cream   1/4 cup sifted unsweeted cocoa
1/2 cup confectioners' sugar   1/2 teaspoon vanilla

1. Combine all ingredients in medium bowl. Refrigerate, covered, 30 minutes.
2. With portable electric mixter at high speed, beat mixture until stiff. Refrigerate until ready to use.

QUESTIONS

1. Why are souffles and baked custards cooked in a pan of water?

2. Explain the effect of overbeating a foam for a souffle.

3. What precautions are necessary when eggs are combined with a hot mixture?

4. Why should egg whites be used immediately after they are beaten?

V. MISCELLANEOUS EGG COOKERY

A. MANICOTTI

Crepe Batter   Cheese Filling
6 large eggs   2 pounds low-fat (skim) ricotta cheese
3/4 cup water   1/2 cup grated Parmesan cheese
3/4 cup milk   2 eggs or egg substitute equivalent
1 1/2 cups all-purpose flour   2 tablespoons chopped parsley
1/4 teaspoon salt   dash salt and pepper

1. Prepare crepe batter:
    a. In a large bowl combine flour, salt, eggs, water, and milk.
    b. With a mixer, blend all ingredients until smooth.
    c. Allow batter to "rest" 30 minutes.
2. Prepare cheese filling:
    a. Mix all ingredients in a medium size bowl.
    b. Refrigerate until ready to use.
3. Making manicotti shells:
    a. Take an 8 inch non-stick omelet pan and rub it with vegetable oil.
    b. Heat omelet pan over medium heat.
    c. Measure out 3 tablespoons of batter into individual custard cups.
    d. Test hotness of pan by sprinkling with water: water should "dance" on surface of pan.
    e. Quickly pour in batter and rotate pan to evenly distribute batter.
    f. Crepe is ready when it feels dry and pulls away from side of pan.
    g. Place each crepe on a piece of wax paper.
    h. Continue making crepes until batter is finished (approximately 16-18 crepes).
4. Assembling crepes:
    a. Spread 1/4 cup of cheese filling down center of each crepe. Roll up and place on a $13 \times 9 \times 2$ inch pan seam side down.
    b. The pan should have some tomato sauce on the bottom. Spoon balance of sauce over top. Sprinkle with grated cheese.
    c. Cover with foil and bake at 375°F for 30 minutes.
    d. Remove foil and bake for another 10 minutes.

QUESTIONS

1. What is the difference between a crepe and a pancake?

2. What is the functional role of the egg in the crepe batter?

3. a. What is meant by a "seasoned pan"?

    b. How does this type of pan affect egg cookery?

LABORATORY 13

Milk and Cheese

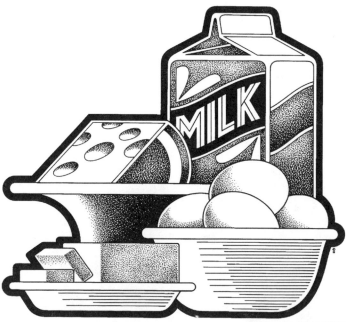

LABORATORY 13
MILK AND CHEESE

Milk is homogenized and pasteurized. There are a variety of milk products available to the consumer. However, the main proteins in these milk products are casein and whey. These proteins affect the cooking quality of milk. Cheese is made from milk. This laboratory exercise will introduce the student to the different types of milk and cheese products as well as their role in food preparation.

VOCABULARY

casein	enzyme	pasteurization	sweet acidophilus milk
Cheddar	evaporated milk	processed cheese	sweetened condensed milk
cheese food	homogenization	rennin	unripened cheese
cheese spread	lactalbumin	ripened cheese	whey
curd	lactoglobulin	soft cheese	

OBJECTIVES

1. To understand how the different proteins found in milk are affected by heat and acid.
2. To become familiar with the different milk and cheese products available.
3. To observe some factors of how milk and cheese behave during cooking.

PRINCIPLES

1. Casein makes up about 80 percent of the protein in milk, while whey makes up the other 20 percent.
2. Whey proteins are made up of lactalbumin and lactoglobulin.
3. Homogenization breaks the fat globules in milk into very small particles that remain dispersed evenly throughout the milk.
4. When milk is heated on a surface unit or range, the whey proteins precipitate and settle on the bottom of the pan.
5. Casein is precipitated by acid. Precipitation of the casein in milk is desirable in making cheese and cultured milk products.
6. Rennin is an enzyme which also precipitates casein in milk.
7. Specific conditions must be met for the rennin precipitation of casein:
   a. active at 104-108°F (40-42°C).
   b. inactivated above 140°F (60°C).
   c. optimal pH 5.8-6.4.
   d. free calcium ions from milk are required by the enzyme to precipitate the casein.
8. In the commercial production of cheese:
   a. a combination of acid and rennin precipitation is used.
   b. pasteurized milk, cream, non-fat milk, or combination are warmed and inoculated with the desired lactic acid producing bacteria.
   c. after sufficient acid has been produced to yield a pH of 5.8, milk is inoculated with rennin.
   d. causes the milk to clot or gel.
   e. the gel is cut into pieces.
   f. then heated slightly to shrink the curd and expel the whey.
   g. the whey is then separated from the curds.
9. Unripened cheese is made of curds with no other treatment except for the addition of a small amount of salt and sometimes cream.
10. Ripened cheese is made of curds that are inoculated with the desired bacteria or mold that gives the cheese its characteristic flavor and texture.
11. Processed cheese is a blend of one or more natural cheeses that have been heated or pasteurized. Emulsifiers and water are added, and the mixture is whipped to form a smooth, homogeneous product. Cheese food and cheese spread are made by the same method as processed cheese; however, they have less fat and more moisture, respectively.

12. When hard cheeses, such as cheddar, Swiss, or Monterey Jack, are heated, they first soften as the fat melts; the higher the fat content, the more readily the cheese liquifies. Continued heating at too high a temperature or for too long a time causes the cheese to lose moisture, shrink, and toughen.
13. Processed cheese is more stable to heat than natural cheese. The emulsifiers in processed cheese improve its blending properties.

I. TO BECOME FAMILIAR WITH VARIOUS AVAILABLE MILK PRODUCTS

A. EVALUATE VARIOUS MILK AND MILK PRODUCTS

Instructions: Various milk and milk products have been selected for evaluation. Please sample the various products in the cups provided and record your observations in the table below.

TABLE FOR EVALUATION OF MILK AND MILK PRODUCTS			
Milk	Appearance	Flavor	Acceptability

II. TO SHOW THE EFFECTS OF TEMPERATURE UPON THE CLOTTING OF MILK BY RENNIN

A.

Temperature	Amount of Milk
42°F	1/2 cup
105°F	1/2 cup
212°F	1/2 cup

1. Adjust temperature of 1/2 cup of milk to each of the stated temperatures.
2. Dissolve 1/4 tablet of rennet in 1 tablespoon of cold water.
3. Add rennet solution to milk. Stir quickly.
4. Allow it to stand at room temperature for 10 minutes.
5. Refrigerate for 1 hour and record results in the table provided.

TABLE FOR OBSERVATIONS OF MILK CLOTTING BY RENNIN	
Temperature	Observation of Formed Clot
42°F	
105°F	
212°F	

QUESTIONS

1. What is the optimum temperature for the coagulation of milk by rennin?

2. What is the reaction involved?

3. List the requirements for the precipitation of casein by rennin.

III. TO STUDY THE EFFECTS OF HEAT AND ACID ON MILK PROTEINS

A. COAGULATION OF MILK BY HEAT

1. Place 1/2 cup milk in small saucepan; place over low heat.
2. Heat slowly to 212°F (100°C). Do not stir. Remove from heat.
3. Record observations in table provided.

B. COAGULATION OF MILK BY ACID

1. Place 1 cup of milk minus 1 tablespoon in a glass measuring cup.
2. Measure the pH: _____.
3. Add 1 tablespoon of vinegar. Stir. Let stand for 5 minutes.
4. Measure the pH: _____.
5. Record observations in table provided.

C. COAGULATION OF SWEETENED CONDENSED MILK BY HEAT

1. Pour 1 can (14 ounces) sweetened condensed milk into an 8 inch or 9 inch pie plate. Cover pie plate with aluminum foil.
2. Pour about 1/4 inch hot water in a larger shallow pan. Place covered pie plate in pan.
3. Bake at 425°F for 1 hour and 20 minutes or until condensed milk is thick and caramel colored (add hot water to pan as needed). Remove foil when done and set aside.
4. Record observations in table provided.

D. **COAGULATION OF SWEETENED CONDENSED MILK BY ACID**

1/2 cup sweetened condensed milk   1/4 cup lemon juice

1. Gradually stir lemon juice with sweetened condensed milk.
2. Allow 10 minutes before cutting into it.
3. Record observations in table provided.

TABLE FOR EVALUATION OF EFFECT OF HEAT AND ACID ON MILK PROTEINS				
Milk	Heat	Acid	Appearance	Proteins Affected
Whole Milk		█		
Whole Milk	█			
Sweetened Condensed Milk		█		
Sweetened Condensed Milk	█			

QUESTIONS

1. a. What effect does heat have on milk?

    b. Which protein is affected?

2. a. What effect does acid have on whole milk?

    b. Which protein is found in the watery part?

    c. Which protein is found in the curd?

3. a. What effect did heat and acid have on the sweetened condensed milk product?

    b. Was it the same effect observed with the whole milk product?

    c. Explain if there were differences.

d. What reaction takes place during the browning of sweetened condensed milk?

IV. TO OBSERVE HOW MILK BEHAVES DURING PREPARATION

A. Cream of Tomato Soup

1 tablespoon butter or margarine
1 tablespoon flour
1/4 teaspoon salt
1/2 cup whole milk, skim milk, or half and half
1 tablespoon tomato paste

2/3 cup tomato juice
1 whole peppercorn
1/4 bay leaf
1 onion, thinly sliced

1. Simmer together for 5 minutes the tomato juice, peppercorn, bay leaf, and onion. Strain into glass measuring cup. Add tomato juice to bring to 2/3 cup. Add tomato paste and blend.
2. Make a white sauce by melting the fat in a saucepan, adding the flour and salt, and blend until smooth. Remove from heat.
3. Slowly add the milk to the tomato. Add this mixture to the roux.
4. Return mixture to heat; bring to a boil with constant stirring.
5. Record observations in table provided.

TABLE FOR EVALUATION OF CREAM OF TOMATO SOUP				
Variation	Appearance	Consistency	Color	Flavor
Whole Milk				
Skim Milk				
Half and Half				

QUESTIONS

1. Describe methods to reduce or eliminate curdling of milk mixtures that contain acidic ingredients.

2. What ingredient serves as a stabilizing agent in the soup recipe?

3. What step or steps are important in the recipe to prevent curdling of the soup?

4. What is a desirable consistency for a cream soup?

V. TO DIFFERENTIATE AMONG THE MANY VARIETIES OF CHEESE AVAILABLE

A. <u>Sample varieties of cheese provided and classify them under the appropriate headings and record other information called for in the table</u>

TABLE FOR CLASSIFICATION OF CHEESE VARIETIES						
Classification	Name	Flavor	Texture	Odor	Color	Uses
1. Unripened A. Low-Fat						
B. High-Fat						

2. Ripened
   A. Bacteria
      1. Soft						

2. Semi-Hard						
3. Hard						
B. Mold 1. Soft						
2. Semi-Hard						
3. Processed						
4. Cheese Food or Spread						

VI. TO COMPARE HOW VARIOUS PROCESSED CHEESE PRODUCTS MELT AS COMPARED TO A NATURAL CHEESE PRODUCT

1. Set out 4 slices of bread.
2. Place cheese to be tested on a separate bread slice.
3. Place bread slices on broiler pan and place broiler pan under a pre-heated broiler.

TABLE FOR EVALUATION OF EFFECT OF HEAT ON CHEESE MELTING					
Type of Cheese	Time to Melt	Smoothness	Consistency	Flavor	Observations
Natural					
Processed Cheese					
Processed Cheese Food					
Processed Cheese Spread					

QUESTIONS

1. Account for the differences, if any, in the:

   a. melting time.

   b. smoothness.

   c. consistency.

   d. flavor.

2. Why were there differences in the melted cheese products?

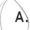

VII. TO UNDERSTAND HOW TO COOK WITH CHEESE

A. MACARONI AND CHEESE

2 cups uncooked elbow macaroni, cooked and drained
   by package directions
1/4 cup flour
1/2 teaspoon salt
1/8 teaspoon white pepper
1/2 teaspoon dry mustard

2 1/2 cups 1 1/2% milk
2 1/2 cups shredded natural Cheddar cheese, mild or
   sharp
1 tablespoon Worcestershire sauce
1 tablespoon finely grated yellow onion

1. Preheat oven to 350°F.
2. Combine together flour, salt, white pepper, and dry mustard in a 2 quart saucepan.
3. Slowly whisk milk into dry ingredients until completely dissolved.
4. Over moderate heat, cook milk mixture, stirring constantly, until thickened.
5. Mix in 2 cups grated Cheddar cheese and all remaining ingredients except macaroni. Cook and stir until cheese melts.
6. Off heat, mix in cooked macaroni; turn mixture into a lightly greased 2 quart casserole, sprinkle top with remaining cheese, and bake uncovered, about 30 minutes, until bubbly and lightly brown.

Variation: Follow the above recipe except substitute either:

1. Low-fat Cheddar cheese
OR
2. Non-fat Cheddar cheese

119

TABLE FOR EVALUATION OF MACARONI AND CHEESE				
Variation	Appearance	Texture	Flavor	Comments
Natural Cheddar Cheese				
Low-fat Cheddar Cheese				
Non-fat Cheddar Cheese				

GENERAL QUESTIONS

1. How is cheese ripened or cured?

2. What determines the fat content of cheese?

3. How is processed cheese prepared?

4. How do cheese food and cheese spread differ from processed cheese?

5. What affect does fat have on the flavor, texture, and the melting property of cheese?

LABORATORY 14

Meat and Poultry

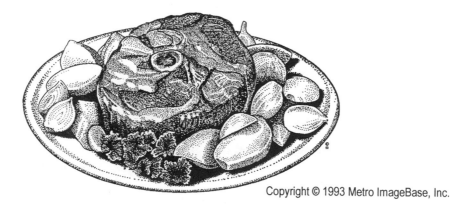

LABORATORY 14
MEAT AND POULTRY

Cooking of a particular cut of meat requires the knowledge of where the piece was derived from the carcass. This will influence whether moist or dry heat should be used. With poultry, however, depending on the age and size of the chicken, either moist or dry heat can be used due to the decreased presence of connective tissue. This laboratory exercise will introduce the student to the selection of different meat cuts and poultry as well as the varied preparation techniques.

VOCABULARY

actin	elastin	marbling	oxymyoglobin
braising	fricassee	muscle fiber	stewing
collagen	gelatin	myoglobin	trichinosis
connective tissue	hemoglobin	myosin	

OBJECTIVES

1. To learn to identify the different cuts of meat and the type of cooking procedures associated with each.
2. To learn the different characteristics between beef, veal, pork, and lamb.
3. To become familiar with organ meats and their preparation.
4. To learn how to disjoint a chicken and the various preparations.

PRINCIPLES

1. The nature and proportions of muscle tissue, connective tissue, and fatty tissue directly affect the eating quality of meats.
2. Muscle fiber is made up of thick filaments composed of myosin protein and thin filaments which make up the actin protein.
3. The connective tissue is made up of collagen which is the principal connective tissue in meat. It is flexible but lacks the degree of elasticity of elastin. Collagen disintegrates into gelatin in hot water while elastin is unaffected.
4. Myoglobin is the pigment in meat that is responsible for its color.
5. Liver, heart, kidney, tongue, brains, sweetbreads, and tripe from various animals are classified as organ or variety meats.
6. Meat can be tenderized by:
   a. grinding.
   b. use of proteolytic enzymes.
   c. by pounding.
   d. by marinating.
   e. by cutting against the grain.
7. The most important reason to cook meat is to make it tender by softening the collagen connective tissues. Excessive heat, however, can actually toughen meat because heat causes the muscle fibers in the lean portion of the muscle to shrink and lose water.
8. Overcooking makes meat tough, rubbery, stringy, and dry. It causes shrinkage of the protein with loss of water from the muscle fibers.
9. Tender cuts of meat can be cooked by dry heat methods: broiling, panbroiling, frying, roasting, and stir-frying.
10. The less tender cuts of meat are cooked by moist heat: braising and stewing.
11. Fully grown chickens are labeled mature chicken, old chicken, hen, stewing chicken, or fowl. Young chickens, in turn, are labeled young chicken, broiler, fryer, roaster, capon, or Rock Cornish game hen.
12. As a rule it is more economical to buy the whole body chicken and cut it as desired.
13. Young poultry has a low content of connective tissue and can be cooked satisfactorily by dry heat methods.
14. Mature birds require long, slow, moist heat cookery to make them tender.
15. When roasting chicken or turkey, an internal temperature of 185°F must be reached.

I. **TO SHOW THE EFFECTS OF THE DEGREE OF DONENESS AS MEASURED BY THE INTERNAL TEMPERATURE AND THE EFFECTS OF ROASTING TEMPERATURE ON THE ROASTING TIME, COOKING LOSSES, AND COLOR AND JUICINESS OF GROUND MEAT PATTIES**

1. Weigh out four 100 gram portions of ground beef.
2. Shape each portion into a round patty of even thickness.
3. To measure the internal temperature, insert short-stemmed or right-angled mercury-filled meat thermometers so that the bulbs are in the center of the patties.
4. Put the meat on a small rack. To catch the drippings, place the rack in a shallow pan for which the weight has been previously recorded.
5. Put 3 samples in an oven at 325°F and roast to the following internal temperatures:
   a. Rare: 130°F (55°C)
   b. Medium: 150°F (65°C)
   c. Well Done: 160°F (71°C)
6. Put one sample in an oven at 425°F and roast to 160°F (71°C).
7. Note and record the roasting time for each. As soon as the meat comes from the oven, remove the thermometer, take the meat from the rack, and weigh. Weigh pans with drippings. Record in the table on next page.
8. With a sharp knife cut each patty in half. Rank samples in descending order for uniformity of doneness.
9. Rank samples in descending order for juiciness in the following table.

QUESTIONS

1. What difference does the roasting temperature make in the

   a. roasting time?

   b. total cooking losses?

   c. uniformity of doneness?

   d. juiciness?

2. Account for the differences observed in the juiciness of the different samples.

3. What are the present standards set for the safe preparation of ground meat?

TABLE FOR EVALUATION OF QUALITY OF COOKED GROUND BEEF

Roasting Temperature °F	Internal Temperature °F	Internal Temperature °C	Cooking Time minute	Raw Weight gm	Cooked Weight gm	% Cooking* Loss gm	% Cooking* Loss %	Pan and Drippings gm	Pan gm	Drippings gm	Evaporation gm	Uniformity of Doneness	Juice
325	130	55											
325	150	65											
325	160	71											
425	160	71											

$$* \text{ \% Cooking Loss} = \frac{\text{Raw Weight (g)} - \text{Cooked Weight(g)}}{\text{Raw Weight (g)}} \times 100$$

II. TO SHOW THE EFFECT OF HEAT AND TREATMENT ON THE COOKING OF LESS TENDER CUTS OF BEEF

SWISS STEAK

8 ounces boneless round steak
dash black pepper
1/4 teaspoon salt
1 tablespoon vegetable oil

1 small onion, sliced
1 can (14 ounces) whole or diced tomatoes with liquid
1 tablespoon flour
1/4 cup water

1. Trim excess fat from steak.
2. Season steak with salt and pepper.
3. Brown steak in hot oil in a skillet; add onions and cook onions with meat until they are tender.
4. Pour tomatoes over meat. Cover pan and simmer approximately 45 minutes. Add more water as needed to keep from burning.
5. Combine flour and 1/4 cup water. Stir into meat; bring mixture to a boil.
6. Evaluate each treatment for tenderness and juiciness.

TREATMENTS

1. Control: Follow directions for Swiss Steak.
2. Pounding: Pound meat with mallet to 1/4 inch thick. Proceed with Swiss Steak recipe.
3. Cutting: Make diagonal slices on both sides of meat, not cutting through. Proceed with Swiss Steak recipe.
4. Enzyme: Sprinkle both sides of meat with commercial enzyme mixture. Proceed with Swiss Steak recipe.
5. Marinade: Marinate meat in 1/2 cup vinegar, 1/4 teaspoon onion powder, and 1/4 teaspoon salt for 15 minutes. Proceed with Swiss Steak recipe.

TABLE FOR EVALUATION OF SWISS STEAK			
Treatment	Tenderness	Juiciness	Appearance of Grain
Control			
Pounding			
Cutting			
Enzyme			
Marinade			

QUESTIONS

1. What procedure yielded the most tender cooked meat?

2. What procedure yielded the juiciest cooked meat?

3. What do you call this type of cooking procedure?

4. How is it different than stewing?

5. Which treatment required a longer cooking time?

6. In the marinade, what ingredient helps in tenderizing?

7. Describe the use and limitations of proteolytic enzymes in increasing the tenderness of meat.

III. TO LEARN TO APPLY DIFFERENT COOKING TECHNIQUES FOR DIFFERENT MEAT CUTS OR VARIETIES

A. BEEF

1. STIR-FRY BEEF

Marinade:
4 tablespoons low sodium soy sauce
1 tablespoon sugar
2 tablespoons dry sherry
1/2-3/4 teaspoon ground ginger
2 garlic cloves, minced

1 pound sirloin, partially frozen

2 tablespoons vegetable oil
1 teaspoon sesame seed oil
1 red pepper, cut into thin strips
1 cup fresh mushrooms, sliced
1/2 head broccoli, cut into flowerets
1 regular onion, cut into 1/8's
1 can (8 ounces) sliced water chestnuts, drained
1/2 cup water
1 tablespoon cornstarch

1. Prepare marinade in a 1 quart bowl.
2. Slice meat into thin strips and place in marinade. Allow meat to marinate at least 30 minutes or longer.
3. Prepare vegetables. Slice peppers into thin strips. Slice mushrooms at least 1/8-1/4 inch thickness. Prepare broccoli into flowerets. Cut onion into wedges.
4. Heat 1 tablespoon vegetable oil and 1 teaspoon sesame seed oil in a 10 inch skillet or wok.
5. Add vegetables and stir-fry 5 minutes or until crisp tender. Remove vegetables.
6. Drain marinade from meat. Add 1 tablespoon oil to skillet. Add meat and stir-fry until no longer pink. Add reserved marinade, stir-fried vegetables, and water chestnuts to skillet and heat all ingredients throughout.
7. Combine 1/2 cup water plus 1 tablespoon cornstarch. Add to skillet, stirring constantly. Cook until mixture thickens and comes to a boil.
8. Serve over cooked rice.

2. BEEF-STUFFED PEPPERS

4 large green peppers
1 pound ground beef
1 medium onion, chopped
2 1/2 cups canned marinara sauce, heated
1 cup cooked rice

1 can (8 3/4 ounces) whole kernel corn, drained
2 teaspoons chili powder
1/2 teaspoon salt
1/2 cup (2 ounces) low-fat Cheddar cheese, shredded

1. Cut off tops of green peppers; remove centers and discard. Cook peppers 5 minutes in boiling water; drain peppers and set aside.
2. Cook ground beef and onion in a large skillet until meat is browned, stirring to crumble meat; drain well.
3. Stir in 1 cup marinara sauce and next 4 ingredients.
4. Stuff peppers with meat mixture, and place in a baking dish. Pour in balance of sauce so it surrounds peppers.
5. Bake at 350°F for 25 minutes. Sprinkle tops of peppers with cheese; bake an additional 5 minutes.

3. SLOPPY JOES

2 teaspoons oil
1 medium onion, coarsely chopped
1 green pepper, diced
3 cloves garlic, minced
1 pound lean chopped meat
1/2 cup ketchup
3/4 cup chili sauce
1 tablespoon tomato paste

1/3 cup water
1 1/2 teaspoons Worcestershire sauce
1 tablespoon chili powder
1 tablespoon cumin
1/2 teaspoon salt
1/4 teaspoon pepper
3 drops hot sauce
4 hamburger buns, split

1. In a large skillet, heat oil. Add onion, green pepper, and garlic.
2. Cook over medium heat until pepper and onion are soft.
3. Add chopped meat. Break up meat until it is crumbly, and browned.
4. Add remaining ingredients, except hamburger buns.
5. Stir until thoroughly combined, and mixture comes to a boil.
6. Lower heat and cover. Cook for 15 minutes.
7. Split hamburger buns in half. Serve hamburger mixture over the buns.

B.) PORK

SWEET AND SOUR PORK
(Reprinted with permission from Betty Crocker's *All Time Favorites*, General Mills, Inc.)

2 pounds pork shoulder
1/3 cup all-purpose flour
2 teaspoons ginger
1/4 cup salad oil
1 can (15 1/2 ounces) pineapple chunks, drained
    (reserve syrup)
1/4 cup vinegar
1/4 cup soy sauce
2 teaspoons Worcestershire sauce

1/3 cup sugar
1 teaspoon salt
1/4 teaspoon black pepper
1 small green pepper, cut into strips
1 can (8 ounces) bean sprouts, drained
1 can (8 ounces) water chestnuts, drained and thinly
    sliced
1 tablespoon chili sauce
cooked rice

1. Cut meat into 1 inch cubes, trimming off any excess fat. Mix half of the flour with the ginger; coat meat thoroughly with the flour mixture.
2. Heat oil in a large skillet or Dutch oven and brown meat, about a third at a time, over medium heat. Remove meat and set aside.
3. Add enough water to the reserved pineapple syrup to make 1 cup and gradually stir in the remaining flour.
4. Stir pineapple syrup mixture, vinegar, soy sauce, and Worcestershire sauce into the fat in the skillet.
5. Heat to boiling, stirring constantly. Boil and stir 1 minute. Stir in sugar, salt, pepper, and meat. Reduce heat. Cover and simmer until the meat is tender, about 1 hour, stirring occasionally.
6. Add pineapple and green pepper and cook 10 minutes. Stir in bean sprouts, water chestnuts, and chili sauce; heat thoroughly, about 5 minutes. Serve over hot rice.

C. LAMB

LAMB CURRY

1 pound boneless lamb shoulder
1 teaspoon salt
1 garlic clove, small
1 large onion
1 cup celery, diced

2 tablespoons vegetable oil
1/2-1 teaspoon curry powder
1 medium apple, tart
cooked rice

1. Cut the meat into 1 inch cubes. Trim away excess fat while cubing.
2. Place the cubed lamb in a saucepan; barely cover with water and add salt; cover and simmer approximately 1 hour.
3. Clean onion, slice into 1/4 inch thick slices. Clean celery and dice. Clean garlic; impale with a toothpick. Add these vegetables to the vegetable oil; cook for 5 minutes. Remove garlic clove.
4. While the onion-celery mixture is cooking, wash, pare, core, and finely chop the apple. Add to the onion-celery mixture; add the curry powder (add the smaller amount first - then add as desired). Add the lamb with whatever liquid remains on the lamb. Simmer uncovered for approximately 20 minutes (mixture can be covered if no excess water is on the lamb).
5. Serve over cooked rice.

D. VARIETY (ORGAN) MEAT

SAUTEED CALF'S LIVER

4 slices turkey bacon
1/3 cup all-purpose flour
1/2 teaspoon salt
1/4 teaspoon black pepper
3/4 pound beef liver, thinly sliced
1 small onion, chopped

2 tablespoons fresh parsley, chopped
2 tablespoons butter or margarine, melted
1 tablespoon lemon juice
pinch of nutmeg
pinch of savory

1. Cook bacon in a large skillet until crisp; remove bacon, reserving the drippings in skillet. Drain and crumble bacon, and set aside.
2. Combine flour, salt, and pepper; dredge liver in flour mixture and brown in reserved bacon drippings plus butter. Remove liver to a warm platter and top with crumbled bacon.
3. Saute onion and parsley in butter; stir in lemon juice, nutmeg, and savory; pour over liver.

QUESTIONS

1. What cuts of meat are suitable for roasting?

2. What is the most accurate way of measuring degree of doneness in meat?

3. Explain how collagen and muscle fibers in meats are affected by heat, and how cooking time and temperature should be controlled for best eating quality.

4. To what temperature should pork be cooked and why?

5. How should variety meats be cooked?

IV. TO OBSERVE AND LEARN HOW TO CUT UP OR DISJOINT A WHOLE CHICKEN

A. DEMONSTRATE HOW TO CUT UP OR DISJOINT CHICKEN

1. Cut the skin parallel to the fold between the thigh and the body cavity of the bird.
2. Grasp the body of the chicken in the left hand and the leg and thigh in the right hand, and bend the latter back until the joint snaps. Cut the thigh muscle from the back as close to the back as possible.
3. To separate the leg from the thigh, bend to locate the joint. Then cut at the joint between leg and thigh. When half way through, reverse direction and cut.
4. Detach wing from the body at the joint.
5. Separate back from ribs.
6. Cut sternum or breast bone from ribs.

V. TO LEARN VARIOUS METHODS FOR CHICKEN PREPARATION

A. CHICKEN AND DUMPLINGS

1/2 cup all-purpose flour	1 cup water
1 1/2 teaspoons salt	pinch of thyme and rosemary
2 teaspoons paprika	1 onion, chopped
1/4 teaspoon black pepper	3 tablespoons all-purpose flour
2 1/4-3 pound broiler fryer	milk
shortening or vegetable oil	Rosemary and Chive Dumplings (below)

1. Mix 1/2 cup flour, salt, paprika, and pepper. Coat chicken with flour mixture.
2. Heat a thin layer of shortening in 12 inch skillet or Dutch oven until hot.
3. Cook chicken in shortening until brown on all sides. Drain fat from skillet; reserve. Add water, onion, and pinch of rosemary and thyme.
4. Cover and cook over low heat until chicken is tender, 45 minutes.
5. Remove chicken from skillet. Remove chicken from bones. Keep chicken in large meaty chunks. Heat 3 tablespoons of reserved fat in skillet. Stir in 3 tablespoons flour. Cook over low heat until mixture is smooth and bubbly.
6. Add enough milk to reserved liquid to measure 3 cups; pour into skillet. Heat to boiling, stirring constantly. Boil and stir 1 minute. Return chicken to gravy.
7. Prepare Rosemary and Chive Dumplings; drop by spoonfuls on hot chicken. Cook, uncovered, 10 minutes, cover and cook 20 minutes longer.

Rosemary and Chive Dumplings

3 tablespoons chives	2 teaspoons baking powder
1 teaspoon dried rosemary, crumbled	3/4 teaspoon salt
3 tablespoons shortening	3/4 cup milk
1 1/2 cups all-purpose flour	

1. Mix together chives, rosemary, flour, salt, and baking powder. Cut in shortening with pastry blender.

129

2. Stir in milk, just until ingredients are combined.
3. Drop by spoonfuls onto hot chicken. Proceed as in step 7 in the above.

B. STIR-FRY CHICKEN

Use Stir-Fry Beef Recipe except:

1. Substitute 1 pound skinless, boneless chicken breast, thinly sliced, for beef.
2. Substitute 1/2 cup chicken broth for 1/2 cup water.
3. Proceed as the recipe indicates.

C. OVEN BARBECUED CHICKEN

3 pounds of chicken pieces

1/2 cup flour
1 teaspoon salt

1/4 teaspoon black pepper
1/4 cup margarine, melted
Texas Barbecue Sauce (below)

1. Preheat oven to 425°F. Spray a 13 × 9 × 2 inch pan with vegetable spray, and set aside.
2. Mix together flour, salt, and pepper. Toss chicken pieces to coat.
3. Place coated chicken pieces in pan, spoon melted margarine evenly over pieces. Bake for 30 minutes.
4. Turn pieces over. Add half of Texas Barbecue Sauce over cooked chicken.
5. Baste chicken with remaining sauce. Bake another 30 minutes or until tender.

Texas Barbecue Sauce

1 tablespoon sugar
1 tablespoon dark brown sugar
1 tablespoon paprika
1 teaspoon salt
1 teaspoon dry mustard
1/4 teaspoon chili powder
1/2 medium onion, chopped

1 cup tomato sauce
1/2 cup water
1/4 cup catsup
1 1/2 tablespoons Worcestershire sauce
1/4 cup cider vinegar
1/8 teaspoon cayenne pepper

1. Mix all ingredients in a saucepan. Simmer, covered, for 15 minutes.

D. CHILI CON CARNE

nonstick cooking spray
2 teaspoons vegetable oil
1 1/4 pounds ground turkey or ground chicken
1 large yellow onion, chopped fine
1/2 medium green pepper, cored, seeded, and chopped
1/2 medium sweet red pepper, cored, seeded, and
    chopped
2 stalks celery, chopped
2 garlic cloves, minced
1 tablespoon chili powder

2 teaspoons ground cumin
1 can (10 1/4 ounces) tomato puree
1 cup hot water plus 1 beef bouillon cube
2 tablespoons tomato paste
1/4 teaspoon red pepper flakes
1 teaspoon ground coriander
1 teaspoon dried oregano, crumbled
1 teaspoon basil, crumbled
1 bay leaf
1 can (15 ounces) red kidney beans, undrained

1. Lightly coat a heavy 10 inch skillet with the cooking spray and set over moderate heat for 30 seconds. Add the ground turkey; cook, stirring often, until no longer pink - about 4-5 minutes. Add the vegetable oil.

130

2. Add the onion, green and red pepper, celery, garlic, chili powder, and cumin; cook until vegetables are soft - about 5 minutes. Add the tomato puree, beef broth, tomato paste, red pepper flakes, coriander, oregano, basil, and bay leaf; simmer, partially covered for 20 minutes, stirring occasionally.
3. Add the kidney beans and simmer, partially covered, 5 minutes longer, stirring occasionally. Discard the bay leaf. Can be served over cooked rice.

E. CHICKEN THIGHS PARADISE

Ginger-Honey Glaze:
1/2 cup orange juice
1/2 teaspoon shredded orange peel
1/4 cup soy sauce
1 tablespoon fresh ginger, pared and chopped
1 tablespoon sugar
1 tablespoon honey
1 large clove garlic, chopped

1/4 cup sliced green onion
1 1/2 teaspoons cornstarch dissolved in 2 tablespoons water
1 teaspoon white vinegar

1 1/2 pounds skinless chicken thighs
butter, margarine or vegetable oil (for basting chicken)

1. In a saucepan stir together Ginger-Honey Glaze ingredients.
2. Cook and stir until bubbly. Continue cooking, stirring constantly, for 2 minutes.
3. Preheat broiler. Line broiler pan with aluminum foil. Spray rack with nonstick vegetable oil cooking spray.
4. Place chicken meat side down on broiler pan.
5. Broil chicken 5 inches from heat for 7 minutes. Broil about 15-20 minutes longer, brushing occasionally with butter, margarine, or oil.
6. Turn chicken and broil for 5 to 15 minutes more or until tender and no longer pink.
7. During last 5 minutes of cooking, brush with Ginger-Honey Glaze. Heat the remaining glaze; serve with chicken.

QUESTIONS

1. Why can chicken be cooked by various cooking methods?

2. Give instructions for using a thermometer when roasting poultry.

3. Briefly describe what to look for when buying good quality poultry.

4. What are the effects of overcooking poultry?

5. How should poultry be handled when it is brought home from the supermarket?

LABORATORY 15

Fish and Seafood
Cookery

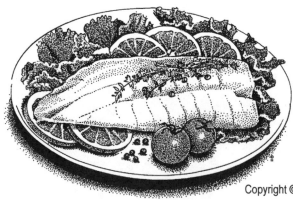

Copyright © 1993 Metro ImageBase, Inc.

LABORATORY 15
FISH AND SEAFOOD COOKERY

Due to a more healthy eating style, people are consuming more seafood. Selection and preparation techniques are required to insure an acceptable product. This laboratory exercise will introduce the student to the proper techniques in selection of quality seafood, and how to preserve these qualities through various preparation techniques.

VOCABULARY

crustaceans	fillet	lean fish
drawn fish	fin fish	mollusks
dressed fish	kippered	roe
fatty fish		

OBJECTIVES

1. To learn how to identify certain market forms of seafood.
2. To learn how to prepare seafood to maintain high quality and nutritional value.

PRINCIPLES

1. Two major categories for the classification of fish are:
   a. vertebrate fish with fins.
   b. shellfish or invertebrates.
2. Shellfish are of two types:
   a. mollusks are soft structure and are either partially or wholly enclosed in a hard shell.
   b. crustaceans are covered with a crustlike shell and have segmented bodies.
3. Examples of mollusks are oysters, clams, abalone, scallops, and mussels. Examples of crustaceans are lobster, crab, shrimp, and crayfish.
4. Fish may be fat or lean. If fat, their oil content is greater than 5%, while lean fish have an oil content of less than 5%. Fat fish tend to be higher in calories and stronger in flavor.
5. High fat fish are lake trout, pompano, salmon, white fish, and catfish.
6. Lean fish are cod, flounder, grouper, haddock, halibut, ocean perch, orange roughy, pike, red snapper, sea bass, sole, and swordfish.
7. There are ways to check for freshness in fish:
   a. eyes are clear and bright.
   b. gills are bright red.
   c. flesh is firm and pliable.
   d. odor is mild with no offensive smell.
8. If fish is frozen it should be packaged tightly wrapped and sealed. It should be solidly frozen and free of ice crystals. Ice crystals indicate fish was thawed and refrozen.
9. The market forms of fish are (FIG.1):
   a. whole.
   b. drawn: entrails are removed.
   c. dressed: head, scales, fins are also removed from a drawn fish.
   d. steaks: taken from a large dressed fish; they are cross-section slices.
   e. fillets: sides of the fish cut lengthwise away from the backbone; they are practically boneless.
10. When cooking fish, choose from baking, broiling, grilling, frying, steaming, and poaching.
11. Dry heat is considered better for cooking fat fish. Lean fish remains moist when cooked by moist heat methods.
12. Fish does not contain connective tissue that is found in meat and poultry and overcooking is a common problem. This will dry and toughen the fish and will, also, destroy the flavor.

13. Check occasionally for doneness while cooking. Pierce the thickest part of the fish. Most fish will flake easily when done, lose its transparency and become opaque.
14. Fish can be cooked in the microwave. Microwave HIGH power to quickly seal in the juices and flavor. Arrange the thicker portion to the outside of the dish so they will get done without overcooking the thinner areas.

Whole or round fish	Dressed or pan-dressed fish	Steaks	Drawn fish	Single fillet

FIG.1. Market forms of fish.

I. TO PREPARE FISH IN A VARIETY OF WAYS

A. BROILED FISH STEAKS

3 fish steaks, 1 inch thick (about 1 pound)   dash of black pepper
1/2 teaspoon salt   2 tablespoons margarine or butter, melted

1. Sprinkle both sides of fish with salt and pepper; brush with half of margarine.
2. Set oven control to broil. Broil with tops about 4 inches from heat until light brown, about 6 minutes; brush fish with margarine.
3. Turn carefully; brush with margarine. Broil until fish flakes very easily with fork and is opaque in center, 4-6 minutes longer.

B. OVEN-FRIED FISH

1 pound fish fillets   1/8 teaspoon garlic powder
2 tablespoons cornmeal   1/8 teaspoon dried dill weed
2 tablespoons dry bread crumbs   dash of black pepper
1 tablespoon Parmesan cheese   2 egg whites, slightly beaten plus 1 tablespoon water
1/4 teaspoon salt   3 tablespoons margarine or butter, melted
1/4 teaspoon paprika

1. Move oven rack to position slightly above middle of oven. Heat oven to 500°F.
2. Cut fish fillets into 2 × 1 1/2 inch pieces.
3. Mix cornmeal, bread crumbs, Parmesan cheese, salt, paprika, dill weed, garlic powder, and pepper. Dip fish into egg white mixture; coat with cornmeal mixture.
4. Place fish in generously greased rectangular pan, 13 × 9 × 2 inches. Pour margarine over fish.
5. Bake uncovered until fish flakes very easily with fork, about 10 minutes.

C. PANFRIED FISH

1 pound fish fillets   1 tablespoon water
1/2 teaspoon salt   1/2 cup all-purpose flour or cornmeal
dash of black pepper   shortening (part margarine or butter)
1 egg

1. If fish fillets are large, cut into serving pieces. Sprinkle both sides of fish with salt and pepper.
2. Beat egg and water until blended. Dip fish into egg then coat with flour.

3. Heat shortening (1/8 inch) in skillet until hot. Fry fish in hot shortening over medium heat, turning fish carefully, until brown on both sides (about 10 minutes).

D. STUFFED-BAKED FISH

1. Prepare stuffing (below).
2. Clean the fish.
3. Lightly salt.
4. Fill with stuffing.
5. Place in a heat resistant platter or dish and bake at 400°F. Allow 10 minutes for each inch of stuffed thickness.

Stuffing for Fish

3 tablespoons minced onion	1/2 teaspoon salt
3/4 cup chopped celery and celery leaves	1/2 teaspoon savory seasoning or thyme
3 tablespoons butter	dash of black pepper
2 cups fresh bread cubes	

1. Cook onion and celery **slowly** in the butter until just tender.
2. Combine all ingredients. **NOTE**: Combine 1 cup of bread for each pound of fish.

QUESTIONS

1. Give directions for cooking fish by:

    a. broiling.

    b. baking.

    c. frying.

    d. steaming.

    e. microwaving.

2. Explain why it is appropriate to cook fish with either dry or moist heat methods.

3. a. Describe typical characteristics of high-quality fresh fish.

135

b.   Suggest appropriate procedures for handling and storing fish and explain why these procedures are necessary.

4.   Why are cooking times different for fish than for meat?

II.   TO LEARN HOW TO PREPARE SHELLFISH

A.   SHRIMP

Shrimp, fresh or frozen (thawed) in the shell

1.   Peel off the shell of fresh or frozen, thawed shrimp.
2.   With a sharp knife, cut along the outside of the center back only deep enough to expose the sand vein.
3.   Remove the sand vein, which may vary in color from light tan to black depending on contents.
4.   Wash the shrimp in running, cold tap water. Hold in cold tap water until it is ready to cook.
5.   Add 3/4 teaspoon salt to each cup of water used for cooking shrimp.
6.   Bring the water to a boil.
7.   Add the cleaned shrimp to the boiling water. Reduce heat.
8.   Cook at simmering temperature, 185-200°F for 5 minutes* or until the meat becomes opaque and some portions of the outer surface become light coral pink.
9.   Drain. Put the shrimp into ice water to chill if they are to be served cold.

*To determine the effect of overcooking, leave one or two shrimp in the cooking water and boil (212°F) these shrimp for 10 minutes. Observe the shrinkage during the cooking period. Compare with the simmered shrimp for tenderness.

1.   Shrimp Scampi

2 pounds medium fresh shrimp
1/4 cup parsley, chopped
4 garlic cloves, crushed
2 tablespoons butter or margarine, melted
2 tablespoons olive oil

1/4 cup dry white wine or vermouth
4 tablespoons lemon juice
1 teaspoon salt
1/4 teaspoon black pepper, freshly ground

1.   Peel and devein shrimp.
2.   Saute parsley and garlic in butter and olive oil until garlic is tender.
3.   Reduce heat to low; add shrimp. Cook, stirring frequently, 2-5 minutes.
4.   Remove shrimp with a slotted spoon to a serving dish; keep warm.
5.   Add remaining ingredients to butter mixture; simmer 2 minutes; pour butter mixture over shrimp.

2.   Spicy Shrimp Creole

1 1/2 pounds fresh shrimp, unpeeled
1 small onion, chopped
1 small green pepper, chopped
1/2 cup celery, chopped
2 medium garlic cloves, minced
2 tablespoons butter or margarine, melted
2 slices turkey bacon, cut into 1/4 inch pieces
1 can (16 ounces) whole tomatoes, undrained and chopped

1 can (8 ounces) tomato sauce
1 tablespoon lemon juice
1 tablespoon brown sugar
2 teaspoons Worcestershire sauce
1/2 teaspoon dried whole thyme
1/8 teaspoon red pepper
1 bay leaf
hot cooked white rice

1. Peel and devein shrimp.
2. Saute onion, green pepper, celery, garlic, and turkey bacon in butter in a Dutch oven until tender.
3. Stir in tomatoes, tomato sauce, lemon juice, brown sugar, Worcestershire sauce, thyme, red pepper, and bay leaf.
4. Cook over medium heat, stirring occasionally, about 30 minutes or until desired consistency.
5. Stir in shrimp and simmer over medium heat 5-10 minutes or until shrimp are done. Serve over rice.

3. Stir-Fried Shrimp With Vegetables

1 pound medium fresh shrimp, unpeeled
1/2 teaspoon salt
1 teaspoon sesame or vegetable oil
1 cup water
3 tablespoons oyster sauce
2 teaspoons cornstarch
1 teaspoon chicken bouillon granules
1/4 cup peanut or vegetable oil
2 cloves garlic, crushed

2 teaspoons fresh ginger root, grated
1 medium sweet red pepper, cored, seeded, minced
1 can (4 ounces) water chestnuts, drained, sliced thin
2 cups diced celery
1/2 pound fresh mushrooms, wiped clean, sliced thin
8 scallions, trimmed, minced
1/2 pound fresh snow pea pods or 1 package (6 ounces) frozen snow pea pods, thawed
2 teaspoons rice wine or white wine

1. Peel and devein shrimp. Sprinkle shrimp with salt; and toss with sesame oil.
2. Combine water, oyster sauce, cornstarch, and bouillon granules; stir well. Set mixture aside.
3. Pour peanut oil around top of preheated wok, coating sides. Allow to heat for 1 minute.
4. Add garlic and ginger root and stir-fry 30 seconds. Add shrimp and stir-fry for 1 1/2 minutes. Remove and drain on paper towels.
5. Add red pepper, water chestnuts, mushrooms, celery, and scallions to wok. Stir-fry 2 minutes. Add pea pods; stir-fry 30 seconds. Add broth mixture, stir-fry constantly until slightly thickened.
6. Stir in shrimp and rice wine. Serve immediately over boiled rice or thin noodles.

QUESTIONS

1. What would contribute to the toughness and shrinkage of the shrimp?

2. How do the methods for simmering a piece of fish and a cut of beef differ?

B. SCALLOPS

BROILED GINGER SCALLOPS

1 pound scallops
1/4 cup soy sauce
1/2 teaspoon minced garlic
2 tablespoons ginger root, finely chopped
2 tablespoons sherry

2 tablespoons lemon juice
1 tablespoon vegetable oil
1/2 teaspoon sesame oil (optional)
1 tablespoon honey

1. If scallops are large, cut into halves. Arrange scallops in single layer in 8 x 8 x 2 inch square baking dish.
2. Heat soy sauce to boiling. Add ginger root and garlic; reduce heat. Simmer, uncovered, 3 minutes. Stir in remaining ingredients; pour over scallops. Cover and refrigerate, stirring occasionally, for 2 hours.

3. Set oven control to broil. Remove scallops from marinade with slotted spoon. Arrange in single layer on rack in broiler pan.
4. Broil with tops 3-4 inches from heat until opaque in center, about 5 minutes. Brush frequently with marinade.

C. SEAFOOD ANALOGS (CRAB, LOBSTER, OR SCALLOPS)

SEAFOOD NEWBURG (Low Fat)

4 teaspoons flour	2 teaspoons margarine
1 1/2 cups skim milk	3 green onions with tops, sliced
2 tablespoons white wine or sherry	1 package (8 ounces) seafood analogs (crabmeat, lobster, or scallops)
1/2 teaspoon salt	paprika
1/2 teaspoon dry mustard	2 tablespoons Romano or Parmesan cheese, grated
4 ounces fresh mushrooms, sliced	7 ounces cooked pasta (linguini, fettucini)

1. In a 1 1/2 quart sauce pan, mix with a wire wisk the flour and milk together. It is important that all the flour is dissolved.
2. Add the wine, salt, and dry mustard.
3. Cook over medium heat, stirring constantly until mixture boils; boil and stir for 1 minute.
4. In an 8 inch or 9 inch nonstick skillet, melt margarine. Add mushrooms and green onion. Stir-fry over medium heat until mushrooms are softened. Season to taste with some salt and pepper.
5. Add cooked mushrooms and seafood analogs to cream sauce. Bring back to a boil.
6. Place sauce in a pie pan. Sprinkle with Parmesan cheese and paprika. Place under broiler and broil until mixture is bubbly.
7. Remove from heat source and serve immediately over cooked pasta.

D. ACCOMPANYING SAUCES

1. COCKTAIL SAUCE

2 tablespoons catsup	1 teaspoon horseradish
1 tablespoon lemon juice	1/4 teaspoon Worcestershire sauce
1/4 teaspoon salt	1-2 drops tabasco

1. Blend together all ingredients.
2. Chill for best flavor.
3. Serve as accompaniment to cooked shrimp.

2. TARTAR SAUCE

1/3 cup mayonnaise	1/2 teaspoon green onion, minced
2 teaspoons sour cucumber pickles, minced	1/2 teaspoon parsley, minced
2 teaspoons green olives, minced	1/2 teaspoon tarragon vinegar
1/2 teaspoon capers	

1. Mix all ingredients together.
2. Serve cold as an accompaniment to fried fish.

3. DRAWN BUTTER SAUCE

3 tablespoons butter or margarine	few grains cayenne pepper
1 1/2 tablespoons flour	1 cup water, boiling
1/4 teaspoon salt	

1. Melt 2 tablespoons of the fat in the upper part of the double boiler.
2. Add the flour; stir until well blended.
3. Add the boiling water gradually; stir until smooth after each addition of water.
4. Bring to a boil over direct heat with continuous stirring.
5. Stir in the remaining butter just before serving. Add salt and cayenne pepper. Serve hot.

GENERAL QUESTIONS

1. What recommendations should be given when cooking shellfish?

2. How important are sanitary conditions when preparing seafood, especially shellfish?

3. What are the nutritional consequences in eating:

   a. finfish?

   b. shellfish?

4. What is the shelf life of fresh fish? How can it be extended?

LABORATORY 16

Legumes and Tofu

LABORATORY 16
LEGUMES AND TOFU

Legumes are an alternate source of protein as well as complex carbohydrates. Legumes are usually in the dried state, therefore, they contain more protein. Tofu is derived from soybeans. Tofu is also known as bean curd which is made by coagulating soy milk. This laboratory exercise will introduce the student to the basic techniques in the preparation of legumes and tofu.

VOCABULARY

legume   rehydration
lentils   tofu
lima bean

OBJECTIVES

1. To be able to identify various available legumes.
2. To learn how to prepare legumes.
3. To become familiar with tofu and its uses in food preparation.

PRINCIPLES

1. Legumes, besides being sources of incomplete protein, are rich sources of complex carbohydrates, including both starch and nondigestible carbohydrate.
2. Legumes should be sorted by removing pebbles and broken or decayed beans. Then surface soil should be washed off.
3. Legumes are usually soaked in water overnight prior to cooking.
4. Another quick way is to heat the soaked beans for 2 minutes by boiling and then soak for 1 hour prior to cooking. This process hastens the rehydration process.
5. Acid interferes with the softening of legumes during cooking by delaying the softening of the cellulose and by inhibiting the softening of the pectin.
6. If legumes are to be seasoned with an acidic ingredient, such as tomatoes or sweet and sour sauce, the acid should not be added until the beans are tender.
7. Calcium and magnesium ions which are found in hard water combine with pectic substances in legumes to form insoluble complexes giving the legumes a firm, almost woody texture.
8. Addition of 1/8 teaspoon of baking soda per cup of dried beans counteracts the effects of hard water. Excessive baking soda produces an alkaline medium that is destructive to thiamin, a vitamin plentiful in legumes.
9. Tofu is also called bean curd or soybean cake.
10. Like soybean products, tofu is an incomplete protein; its greatest value is in its ability to extend animal proteins.
11. Calcium sulfate provides the greatest volume of tofu, while calcium chloride produces a firmer tofu.
12. Fresh tofu is sold in blocks immersed in water in covered plastic containers.
13. Tofu has a bland flavor which takes up any flavor added.
14. Tofu exhibits a porous texture when it is frozen and then thawed.

I.   TO LEARN HOW TO IDENTIFY AND PREPARE LEGUMES

A.   IDENTIFICATION OF LEGUMES

Selected legumes will be left on a tray. You will examine each one and identify them. Fill in the table provided.

TABLE FOR IDENTIFICATION OF LEGUMES			
Legume	Shape	Color	Description

B. RECIPES WITH LEGUMES

1. CHEESEY LENTILS

2 cups water
6 ounces dried lentils
1 tablespoon instant chicken bouillon
1 medium onion, chopped

1 tablespoon red-wine vinegar
1 medium green pepper, chopped
1/2 cup grated Cheddar or reduced fat cheese
1 medium tomato, chopped

1. Heat water and lentils to boiling in 2 quart saucepan; stir in bouillon (dry).
2. Cover and simmer until lentils are tender, about 30 minutes. Add more water during cooking, if necessary.
3. Stir in onion, vinegar, and green pepper; simmer uncovered 5 minutes.
4. Stir in tomato. Sprinkle with cheese.

2. ITALIAN LIMA BEANS

2 cups water
1/2 pound dried lima beans
1 teaspoon salt
2 tablespoons olive oil
1 cup celery, thinly sliced
1/4 cup Parmesan or Romano cheese, grated

1 cup carrots, thinly sliced
1/2 teaspoon dried basil leaves
1 medium onion, finely chopped
1 medium green pepper, chopped
1 can (8 ounces) tomato sauce

1. Preheat oven to 375°F.
2. Heat water, beans, and salt to boiling in Dutch oven. Boil 2 minutes; remove from heat. Cover and let stand 1 hour.
3. Add enough water to beans to cover, if necessary. Heat to boiling; reduce heat. Cover; simmer until tender; 1 1/4 -1 1/2 hours. Add more water during cooking.
4. Drain beans. Heat the oil in a large skillet; add the chopped onion and pepper; saute for a few minutes.
5. Add the carrots and celery and cook until crisp tender. Add tomato sauce, basil leaves, and Romano or Parmesan cheese. Mix sauce and beans together.
6. Add ingredients to a greased 2 quart casserole. Bake uncovered in a 375°F oven until hot and bubbly, about 25 minutes.

3. WESTERN BEAN STEW

1 cup pinto beans, dry
3 cups water to soak dry beans
1/2 teaspoon salt
2-3 drops Tabasco sauce
2 tablespoons shortening
1 medium onion, chopped

1 small garlic clove, minced
1 cup canned tomatoes
2 tablespoons parsley, minced
1/2 cup water
1/4 teaspoon ground marjoram
1 teaspoon chili powder

1. Sort and wash beans. Soak overnight.
2. Add salt and Tabasco sauce to beans; bring to a boil; reduce heat; simmer until beans are tender, approximately 1 hour. Drain beans.
3. While beans are cooking, melt fat in a heavy frying pan; add onions and garlic; cook until onion is light yellow. Add tomatoes, parsley, 1/2 cup of water, and the spices; simmer together for 30 minutes.
4. Add beans to onion mixture; simmer together for an additional 15 minutes.

4. SPLIT PEA SOUP

1/2 cup split peas
3 cups water
2 ounces smoked ham
1 medium onion, minced
1 clove garlic, peeled, minced

1/2 cup carrot, grated
1 stalk celery, sliced
1/4 teaspoon dry mustard
salt, pepper, paprika

1. Wash peas and combine with all ingredients except the seasonings.
2. Simmer until tender. Sieve, if desired.
3. Add seasoning and garnish with slices of hard-cooked egg or lemon.

5. LENTIL STEW

2 teaspoons vegetable oil
2 medium onions, chopped
1 garlic clove, finely chopped
3 cups water
2 medium potatoes, coarsely chopped
1 cup dried lentils, sorted, rinsed
1/4 cup fresh parsley, chopped
1 bay leaf
1/4 teaspoon coriander

1/4 teaspoon cardamon
1/2 teaspoon ground cumin
1/2 teaspoon salt
1/4 teaspoon pepper
1/8 teaspoon mace
1/8 teaspoon cinnamon
8 ounces small fresh mushrooms, cut in half
1 can (28 ounces) whole tomatoes, undrained

1. Heat oil in Dutch oven over medium heat.
2. Saute onions and garlic in oil.
3. Stir in remaining ingredients; break up tomatoes. Heat to boiling; reduce heat.
4. Cover and simmer about 40 minutes, stirring occasionally, until potatoes are tender.

QUESTIONS

1. For what foods may legumes be substituted in the diet?

2. How do legumes compare with other protein-rich foods in nutritive value?

3. What are the basic principles in cooking legumes?

4. What factors influence the cooking time of legumes?

5. a. What is the test for doneness of legumes?

   b. What would happen if the following were added to legumes before they were fully cooked: tomato sauce; catsup; brown sugar?

II. TO LEARN ABOUT AND BECOME ACQUAINTED WITH TOFU IN FOOD PREPARATION

A. TOFU AND TUNA SALAD

1 can (6 1/2 ounces) tuna
1 1/2 cups tofu, mashed
1 cup celery, chopped
1/2 cup onion, chopped

1/2 teaspoon dill seed
dash of black pepper
1/2 cup mayonnaise

1. Drain tuna thoroughly and flake.
2. Thoroughly mix all ingredients. Chill.

B. TOFU SPINACH PIE

1 9 inch pie shell
1 package (10 ounces) frozen spinach, thawed, chopped
1/3 cup oil
1 1/2 cups onion, chopped

1 pound tofu, crumbled
1 teaspoon garlic powder
1 tablespoon lemon juice
1 1/2 teaspoons salt

1. Preheat oven to 400°F.
2. Partially bake the pie shell (5 minutes). Remove from oven.
3. Steam or boil the spinach and drain well.
4. Saute onions in oil until soft.
5. Add steamed spinach to onions and saute for 2 minutes more.
6. Add crumbled tofu, lemon juice, and garlic powder to spinach mixture.
7. Pour mixture into the partially baked pie shell. Bake for about 30 minutes until crust is golden.

C. CHILI CON TOFU WITH BEANS

1 1/4 cups cooked pinto beans, with liquid
1/2 pound frozen tofu
1 tablespoon soy sauce
1 tablespoon tomato paste
1 cup canned tomatoes
1/2 tablespoon peanut butter
dash of onion powder
dash of garlic powder

2 tablespoons water
2 tablespoons oil
1 large green pepper, diced
1 large onion, diced
1 teaspoon salt
2 1/2 teaspoons chili powder
dash of cumin
1 garlic clove, minced

1. Thaw and squeeze the water out of the frozen tofu. Tear into bite size pieces.
2. Mix together soy sauce, tomato paste, peanut butter, onion powder, garlic powder, water, and 1/2 tablespoon oil. Add tofu to this mixture and mix well until all pieces are evenly coated.
3. Fry tofu mixture in 1 tablespoon oil over medium heat until brown.
4. In a separate pan, heat 1/2 tablespoon oil. Saute onion, green pepper, and garlic until onions are transparent.
5. Add the sauteed vegetables, tomatoes, and beans to the tofu. Add water if needed to cover.
6. Add remaining spices to tofu and bring to a simmer.

QUESTIONS

1. Briefly describe the source and preparation of tofu.

2. What happens to tofu when it is frozen?

3. What types of preparation methods are best suited for soft tofu?

4. What types of preparation methods are best suited for firm tofu?

LABORATORY 17

Sugar Crystallization

LABORATORY 17
SUGAR CRYSTALLIZATION

Candy making is an art which requires accuracy in measuring and cooking. Sugar plays an important role in developing the texture and consistency of candy. Cooking the sugar solution to the proper point will insure a quality product. This laboratory exercise will introduce the student to the different types of candy and the preparation techniques that are used to make the particular varieties.

VOCABULARY

amorphous candy	disaccharide	monosaccharide	seeding
caramelizing sugar	fructose	nuclei sites	sucrose
corn syrup	interfering agent	saturated solution	supersaturated solution
crystalline candy	invert sugar		

OBJECTIVES

1. To better understand the principles involved in the successful preparation of various types of candies.
2. To observe and understand the difference between crystalline candy and amorphous candy.
3. To understand the manipulation of heating, cooling, and beating and the effect they will have on crystalline candy.

PRINCIPLES

1. An invert sugar is a mixture of equal amounts of glucose and fructose resulting from the hydrolysis of sucrose.
2. To make most candies, sucrose solutions are boiled until enough water is evaporated to produce a sugar concentration that yields a candy of the desired consistency.
3. Crystalline candies contain sucrose crystals. Fondant, fudge, panocha, divinity, creams, and nougats are crystalline candies.
4. Crystalline candies have crystals so small that they go undetected by the tongue.
5. In order for the crystals to be small, sucrose must be completely dissolved and must be cooked to the correct concentration.
6. The steps necessary to obtain an acceptable crystalline candy are:
   a. heating: boil the sucrose solution as rapidly as possible in an open pot to evaporate the excess water.
   b. cooling: a **supersaturated** syrup is necessary to produce small crystals in candy. As the syrup cools it becomes more viscous, an effect that favors formation of many small nuclei when crystallization begins.
   c. agitation: once a supersaturated solution is obtained, the viscous syrup must be rapidly beaten to produce numerous small crystals. Beat until dull.
7. Interfering substances in the sugar solution promote supersaturation by inhibiting the formation of crystals. Interfering substances include corn syrup, butter, milk, cream, chocolate, cocoa, gelatin, and egg white. They have a different structure than sucrose and physically interfere with sucrose crystals growing on each other.
8. Noncrystalline candies are also known as amorphous candies because they do not contain crystals. Such candies either contain large amounts of interfering agents or have been cooked to high end-point temperatures evaporating all the water.

ATTENTION

Before beginning to make candy, check the boiling point of the thermometer you are using. Adjust the temperatures in the recipes according to your results. For example, if water boiled at 210°F (99°C), lower temperature given in the recipes by 2°F (1°C)

I. TO SUCCESSFULLY PREPARE CRYSTALLINE CANDY BY LEARNING THE PRINCIPLES OF PROPER MANIPULATION

A. CHOCOLATE FUDGE

2 cups sugar
2/3 cup milk
2 tablespoons light corn syrup
1/4 teaspoon salt

2 ounces unsweetened chocolate
2 tablespoons margarine
1 teaspoon vanilla
1/2 cup nuts, if desired, coarsely chopped

1. Butter loaf pan, 9 × 5 × 3 inches. Cook sugar, milk, corn syrup, salt, and chocolate in a 2 quart saucepan over medium heat, stirring constantly, until chocolate is melted and sugar is dissolved.
2. Cook, stirring occasionally, to 234°F on candy thermometer or until small amount of mixture dropped into very cold water forms a soft ball that flattens when removed from water.
3. Remove from heat. Add margarine. Do not mix.
4. Cool mixture to 120°F without stirring (bottom of saucepan will be lukewarm). Add vanilla.
5. Beat vigorously and continuously 5-10 minutes or until candy is thick and no longer glossy.
6. Quickly stir in nuts. Spread in pan. Cool until firm. Cut into 1 inch squares.

B. PENUCHE

1 cup sugar
1 cup light brown sugar
2/3 cup milk
2 tablespoons light corn syrup

1/4 teaspoon salt
2 tablespoons margarine
1 teaspoon vanilla
1/2 cup nuts, if desired, coarsely chopped

1. Butter loaf pan, 9 × 5 × 3 inches. Cook sugars, milk, corn syrup, and salt in a 2 quart saucepan over medium heat, stirring constantly, until sugars are dissolved.
2. Cook, stirring occasionally, to 234°F on candy thermometer or until small amount of mixture dropped into very cold water forms a soft ball that flattens when removed from water.
3. Remove from heat. Add margarine. Cool mixture to 120°F without stirring.
4. Add vanilla. Beat vigorously and continuously 5-10 minutes or until candy is thick and no longer glossy.
5. Quickly stir in nuts. Spread in pan. Cool until firm. Cut into 1 inch squares.

C. DIVINITY

1 cup sugar
2 tablespoons corn syrup
1/4 cup boiling water

1 egg white
dash of salt
1/2 teaspoon vanilla

1. Mix first three ingredients in a saucepan and stir until the sugar is dissolved, or heat 2-3 minutes in a covered pan.
2. Remove lid and boil rapidly to 252°F (122°C).
3. Add salt to egg white and beat until stiff but still shiny.
4. Pour hot syrup over beaten egg white, beating continuously.
5. Beat until thick and stiff enough to hold its shape and until candy begins to lose its gloss.
6. Add flavoring and drop onto wax paper.

TABLE FOR EVALUATION OF CRYSTALLINE CANDY				
Crystalline Candy	Firmness	Crystal Size	Smoothness	Flavor
Chocolate Fudge				
Penuche				
Divinity				

QUESTIONS

1. What is invert sugar? How is it obtained?

2. Distinguish between a saturated and a supersaturated sugar solution.

3. Describe briefly the procedure required to obtain a supersaturated solution.

4. Why must a supersaturated solution be obtained in making crystalline candies?

5. Why is it necessary to wipe the sides of the pan clear of sugar?

6. Why is it necessary not to jar the pan during the cooling process?

7. What are the interfering agents in candy making and give examples of them found in the candies prepared?

II. TO OBSERVE AND SUCCESSFULLY PREPARE AMORPHOUS CANDY

A. CARAMELS

1 cup sugar, granulated	1/2 cup butter or margarine
1 cup corn syrup, dark	1 teaspoon vanilla extract
1 cup cream, divided	butter to grease pan

1. Check boiling point of water on candy thermometer.
2. Lightly butter the bottom and sides of an 8 × 8 inch pan.
3. Using a 2 quart saucepan, blend together the sugar, corn syrup, butter, and 1/2 cup cream. Bring to a boil, stirring constantly.
4. Cook over moderate heat, stirring constantly to 240°F.
5. Remove from heat and add very gradually the balance of cream (1/2 cup).

6. Return to heat and cook to 244-246°F. Stir in vanilla quickly.
7. Pour the mixture at once, without stirring, into a buttered pan. Allow caramels to set until cool. Loosen from sides of pan with case knife. Invert the candy onto a wooden board.
8. Cut with lightly buttered knife; wrap in waxed paper.

B. PEANUT BRITTLE

1 1/2 cups sugar, granulated
1/2 cup corn syrup, light
1/2 cup water
3 tablespoons butter or margarine

1/2 teaspoon soda
1 1/2 cups roasted peanuts, coarsely chopped
1/2 teaspoon vanilla extract

1. Check boiling point of water on candy thermometer.
2. Use 1 tablespoon of margarine to lightly grease the surface of three large baking sheets (without sides).
3. Using a 2 quart saucepan, combine the water, corn syrup, and sugar in the saucepan. Place the thermometer in position.
4. Heat mixture rapidly to 280°F (138°C). Stir to keep mixture from scorching. It may be desirable to wipe undissolved sugar crystals from the side of the pan with damp cheesecloth wrapped around a fork.
5. When the syrup reaches 280°F (138°C), add the peanuts and the butter or margarine. Stir the mixture continuously and heat to 306°F (152°C). Remove pan from heat immediately. Remember to make temperature adjustments for original thermometer reading for boiling water; if water boiled at 210°F (99°C), cook to 304°F (151°C).
6. Add the soda and the vanilla; stir these ingredients in as quickly as possible. **Do not overstir or the foam structure will be lost**.
7. Pour approximately one third of the final mixture on each of three baking sheets. Pour into as thin a layer as possible, but do not try to spread the mixture with a spatula.
8. After the edges of the candy have cooled slightly - about 2 minutes - start to gently pull and stretch the candy into a relatively thin sheet. Try to keep the nuts fairly evenly distributed during stretching. Continue to stretch the candy until the center of the mass has also been stretched.
9. When completely cool, break into pieces.

C. TOFFEE

1 cup sugar
1/2 cup butter
1/4 cup water

1 tablespoon corn syrup
1/2 cup almonds, blanched, toasted, chopped
1/8 pound of milk chocolate

1. Mix sugar, butter, water, and corn syrup in saucepan and stir until sugar is dissolved.
2. Cook on medium heat to the hard-crack stage (300°F or 149°C), stirring to prevent scorching.
3. Stir in almonds and pour into an oiled, 8 × 8 × 2 inch pan.
4. When candy is cool, spread with chocolate which has been melted in a double boiler over warm (115°F or 46°C) water.
5. When cold, break into pieces.

TABLE FOR EVALUATION OF AMORPHOUS CANDY				
AMORPHOUS CANDY	FIRMNESS	CRYSTAL SIZE	SMOOTHNESS	FLAVOR
Caramels				
Peanut Brittle				
Toffee				

QUESTIONS

1. What interfering agents are used in caramels?

    What is their function?

2. What is the function of baking soda in the peanut brittle?

3. What is the main difference between amorphous and crystalline candies?

4. What determines the consistency of fudge?

    Caramels?

5. What process is responsible for the production of color in:

    a. peanut brittle?

    b. caramels?

LABORATORY 18

Ice Crystallization
(Frozen Desserts)

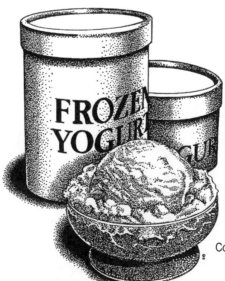

LABORATORY 18
ICE CRYSTALLIZATION (FROZEN DESSERTS)

On a hot summer day, people always look for something cold and refreshing. Ice cream has been a favorite selection for such an occasion. Body and texture are terms used when rating ice cream. Sugar plays a supporting role, along with the other ingredients in the recipe to ensure proper body and texture. The student will learn in this laboratory exercise how the selection and manipulation of the ingredients in the ice cream recipe will enhance body and texture.

VOCABULARY

body	emulsifier	stabilizer	texture
brine	overrun (swell)	still frozen	

OBJECTIVES

1. To understand the functional role of ingredients in an ice cream formulation.
2. To understand how the rate of freezing and manipulation affects the formation of ice crystals.
3. To differentiate between body and texture when describing quality in a frozen dessert.

PRINCIPLES

1. Ingredients in a frozen dessert include liquid from some source and sugar. Optional ingredients include gelatin, eggs, milk solids, emulsifiers, and stabilizers.
2. The ingredients used influence the consistency, texture, and flavor of the frozen dessert.
3. Sugar decreases the freezing point of frozen dessert mixtures, thus interfering with water crystallization.
4. Cream and milk provide fat; the more fat in the mixture the smoother it becomes by interfering with the crystal growth or formation.
5. Emulsifiers are used to keep the fat dispersed and stabilizers are used to keep the other ingredients well distributed. They both function to keep crystal size small and help improve the body of the frozen dessert.
6. Overrun is the increase in volume of a frozen dessert mixture when it is frozen. While part of this increase in volume results from the expansion of the water during freezing, most of it is due to the incorporation of air in the mixture during freezing.
7. Still frozen desserts are not agitated during their freezing, but are whipped after they are partially frozen. They do not have the same texture and body as the agitated frozen dessert, and ice crystals grow faster in these types.

I. PREPARATION OF FREEZER AND FREEZE MIXTURE

1. See that all parts of the freezer fit and are in working order.
2. Scald freezer can and dasher.
3. Pour mixture to be frozen into freeze can. Do not fill more than 2/3-3/4 full.
4. Adjust dasher and lid and place in freezer.
5. Adjust crank before adding ice and salt. Place freezer in a dishpan to catch spills.
6. Fill freezer 1/3 full with ice before adding any salt. Then add salt and ice in layers.
7. Have salt and ice slightly higher than the level of the mix in the freezer can.
8. For ice creams, use 1 part salt to 8 parts ice by weight (1/4 cup salt per quart of ice). Three to four quarts of crushed ice are needed for 1 quart freezer.
9. For ices and sherbets, use 1 part salt to 6 parts ice by weight (1/3 cup of salt per quart crushed ice).

Freezing Process

10. Follow manufacturer's direction for freezing the mixture.

<u>Packing the Dessert</u>

11. Remove dasher and pack down the frozen mixture into another bowl.
12. Cover the surface of the ice cream with a piece of waxed paper.
13. Cover bowl entirely; place in freezer.

<u>Observations</u>

1. Determine the temperature of the mix and of the brine and record it in the table provided (page 156).
2. Determine the **swell** or **overrun** as follows:
    a. measure the depth of the can (A).
    b. measure from top of can to top of mix before freezing (B), subtract to get depth of mix (A - B = C).
    c. as soon as mixture is frozen, remove dasher and measure to top of frozen mix (D).
    d. subtract original depth of mix to get the amount of swell (C - D).
    e. divide the amount of swell by original depth and multiply quotient by 100; this gives percent of swell or overrun.
    f. formula:

$$\% \text{ swell or overrun} = \frac{C - D}{C} \times 100$$

A. VANILLA ICE CREAM

2 egg yolks, beaten
1/2 cup sugar
1/2 teaspoon unflavored gelatin
1 cup milk

1/4 teaspoon salt
2 cups chilled whipping cream
1 tablespoon vanilla

1. Whisk together egg yolks, sugar, gelatin, milk, and salt in the top part of a double boiler.
2. Cook over simmering water until mixture is slightly thickened or coats a spoon.
3. Refrigerate in chilled bowl, 2-3 hours (or chill over ice mixture).
4. Stir whipping cream and vanilla into milk mixture.
5. Pour into freezer can; put dasher in place.
6. Freeze mixture according to manufacturer's instructions.
7. Allow to ripen for several hours before serving.

B. OLD FASHIONED LEMON ICE CREAM

2 cups milk
1/4 teaspoon salt
1 1/2 cups sugar
2 tablespoons + 2 teaspoons flour
2 eggs, separated

1 cup half and half
1 cup whipping cream
2 teaspoons vanilla
1/4 teaspoon grated lemon peel
1/4 cup + 2 tablespoons fresh lemon juice

1. Combine sugar, flour, and salt in a 2 quart saucepan.
2. Gradually add milk; blend until dry ingredients are dissolved.
3. Cook over medium heat, stirring constantly until thickened.
4. Gradually stir in approximately 1/4 of the hot mixture into the 2 beaten egg yolks. Add to remaining hot mixture stirring constantly. Cook 1 minute; remove from heat and let cool. Cover and refrigerate 2-24 hours. (For faster results, place mixture over ice to cool rapidly.)
5. Add half and half, whipping cream, vanilla, and grated lemon peel to the chilled mixture.
6. Pour lemon juice over milk mixture; beat well.
7. Beat egg whites, add to mixture, and blend.
8. Pour mixture into freezer container. Freeze according to manufacturer's instructions.

C. **CHOCOLATE ICE CREAM**

2 cups milk
1/2 teaspoon unflavored gelatin
2 egg yolks
1 cup sugar
2 cups whipping cream

2 teaspoons vanilla
3 ounces semi-sweet chocolate
2 ounces unsweetened chocolate
1/3 cup chocolate chips (optional)

1. Soften gelatin in 1/2 cup milk. Set aside.
2. Scald balance (1 1/2 cups) of milk in the top of a double boiler. Add the softened gelatin.
3. Beat the yolks together with the sugar in a bowl, until they turn light and form a ribbon.
4. Continue beating while slowly pouring the milk into the yolks.
5. Transfer the ingredients back to the saucepan.
6. Cook over simmering water, stirring constantly with a rubber spatula.
7. Heat until the custard coats the spatula.
8. Remove the custard from the heat and mix in 1 cup of the heavy cream and vanilla.
9. Over very low heat, mix together the chocolate and the remaining cream in a small saucepan, until the chocolate has completely melted.
10. Beat into the custard. Cool completely.
11. Freeze according to the manufacturer's instructions.
12. When the ice cream is nearly set, add the chocolate chips.
13. Place in a covered container and harden before serving.

D. **STRAWBERRY ICE CREAM**

1. Follow ingredients and directions for Vanilla Ice Cream except:
   a. decrease vanilla to 1 teaspoon.
   b. stir 1 package (16 ounces) frozen strawberry halves, thawed, into milk mixture after adding vanilla.
   c. stir in few drops red flood color, if desired.

E. **ORANGE SHERBET**

1/2 cup + 2 tablespoons water
1/2 cup milk
1/2 teaspoon unflavored gelatin
1/2 cup sugar

1/2 cup orange juice
1 tablespoon lemon juice
1/2 teaspoon orange rind, grated
dash of salt

1. Hydrate gelatin in 2 tablespoons water.
2. Heat water; add sugar and hydrated gelatin. Stir over heat to dissolve ingredients.
3. Cool and add the remaining ingredients.
4. Freeze according to manufacturer's directions.

NOTE: This recipe needs to be doubled in order to fit into the normal ice cream freezer. If using the smaller hand-cranked models that are placed directly in the freezer, this recipe "as is" would be perfect.

F. **FROZEN VANILLA YOGURT**
(Reprinted with permission of the Meredith Corporation, *Better Homes and Gardens Family Favorites Made Lighter*, 1992, p. 219.)

1 1/2 cups sugar
1 can (12 ounces) skim evaporated milk
1 envelope (1 tablespoon) unflavored gelatin

2 tablespoons vanilla extract
4 containers (8 ounces each) low-fat or non-fat plain yogurt

1. In a 1 1/2 quart sauce pan, mix together sugar and unflavored gelatin.
2. Add skim milk and mix thoroughly. Allow mixture to stand 5 minutes to allow gelatin to soften.
3. Place saucepan on moderate heat and cook, stirring constantly. Bring mixture up to the boiling point. Remove from heat. Cool thoroughly.
4. When the mixture has cooled, add vanilla extract.
5. With a wire whisk, gradually add the yogurt to the cooled gelatin mixture.
6. Freeze mixture according to the manufacturer's instructions.

Variation: During the last 15 minutes of freezing, add 1 cup of fresh peach puree to the frozen mixture.

TABLE FOR EVALUATION OF QUALITY ATTRIBUTES OF FROZEN DESSERTS						
Frozen Dessert Type	Temperature of Brine	Temperature of Mix	% Swell	Body	Texture	Flavor
Vanilla Ice Cream						
Old-Fashioned Lemon Ice Cream						
Chocolate Ice Cream						
Strawberry Ice Cream						
Orange Sherbet						
Frozen Vanilla Yogurt						

QUESTIONS

1. Distinguish between ice cream, ice milk, sherbet, sorbet, and ices.

2. Why is rock salt combined with ice to freeze dessert mixes.

3. Briefly discuss the functions of sugar and fat in frozen dessert mixes.

4. What causes swell or overrun in frozen desserts?

   Why is it important?

5. Why was gelatin used in the various recipes?

6. What is the cause of sandiness in ice cream?

7. What do frozen desserts and crystalline candies have in common?

II. TO USE STILL-FREEZING IN THE MAKING OF FROZEN DESSERTS

A. ITALIAN LEMON ICE

juice of 6 lemons
2 1/2 cups water
1 cup sugar

rind of 1 lemon
1 egg white

1. Squeeze lemons and discard seed.
2. Combine water and sugar in saucepan. Bring to a boil and boil gently for 5 minutes. Cool.
3. Stir in lemon juice and rind. Using a whisk, beat in egg white.
4. Pour mixture into ice cube trays or freeze container.
5. When lemon ice is semi-frozen (2-3 hours) remove from freezer. Transfer to a bowl and beat for 1 minute.
6. Pour back into a container and freeze.

B. CHOCOLATE MOUSSE

1 1/2 cups milk
3 squares (1 ounce each) semisweet chocolate, cut into pieces
1/4 cup sugar
3 eggs, separated

1 teaspoon vanilla
1/2 teaspoon cream of tartar
3/4 cup chilled whipping cream

1. In a saucepan over low heat stir and scald milk, sugar, and chocolate. Heat until chocolate melts.
2. Remove from heat; beat in egg yolks; return custard to low heat and stir constantly until it thickens. Strain mixture. Cool pan over ice. Add vanilla.
3. Beat egg whites and cream of tartar in 2 1/2 quart bowl until stiff, but shiny peaks.
4. Stir about 1/4 of the meringue into chocolate mixture. Fold into remaining meringue.
5. Beat whipping cream until stiff. Fold into chocolate meringue. Spoon into dessert dishes.
6. Refrigerate at least 2 hours, but no longer than 48 hours.

EVALUATION TABLE FOR STILL-FROZEN DESSERTS			
Still Frozen Dessert	Body	Texture	Flavor
Italian Lemon Ice			
Chocolate Mousse			

QUESTIONS

1. What is a mousse?

2. How is air incorporated into still-frozen desserts?

3. How is crystal growth prevented in still-frozen desserts?

LABORATORY 19

Beverages:
Coffee, Tea, and
Cocoa

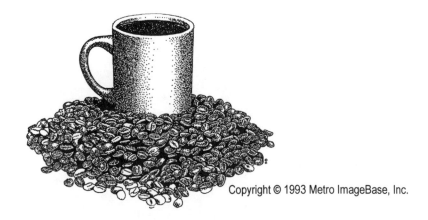

LABORATORY 19
BEVERAGES: COFFEE, TEA, AND COCOA

Coffee, tea, and cocoa are prepared and enjoyed world-wide. Aroma and body are key quality factors that are usually associated with these products. Careful preparation is important in order to enjoy these products to their fullest. This laboratory exercise will introduce the student to the selection of various coffees, teas, and cocoa/chocolate products and the proper preparation of each.

VOCABULARY

black tea	drip method	green tea	percolation
caffeine	Dutch-processed cocoa	natural-processed cocoa	polyphenol
conching	freeze-dried	oolong tea	tannin
decaffeinated			

OBJECTIVES

1. To learn differences between the various coffees, teas, and cocoas available.
2. To emphasize the main factors for success in brewing tea and in making coffee and hot chocolate.

PRINCIPLES

1. Coffee that is available to the consumer is usually a blend of as many as 5 or 6 different varieties of coffee beans.
2. Green coffee beans have little flavor and aroma until **roasted**.
3. Bitterness in coffee becomes more pronounced as the polyphenol content increases. Polyphenol solubility apparently increases with temperature, and a boiling temperature releases polyphenols readily from the coffee bean.
4. Air and moisture decrease the flavor and shelf life of ground coffee.
5. Coffee may be ground:
   a. regular ground which is used for percolated coffee; or
   b. fine ground which contains no coarse particles and is used for drip coffee.
6. 185-203°F (85-95°C) is optimum for brewing a good coffee beverage. Polyphenols are more soluble at boiling and give a bitter product.
7. A clean coffee pot is essential in making a good coffee beverage.
8. Tea is derived from the leaf of an evergreen shrub.
9. Fermentation determines the color and flavor of the tea.
10. There are three varieties of tea:
    a. green tea: leaves are steamed to inactivate the enzymes; then are rolled and dried.
    b. oolong tea: partially fermented tea.
    c. black tea: leaves are withered and rolled to release enzymes for fermentation.
11. Because the polyphenol content of tea is fairly high, excessive steeping, especially at or near the boiling point, extracts more bitter polyphenol substances than is desirable.
12. Cocoa and chocolate are made by grinding the seeds of the cacao tree. To decrease the bitter taste, the seeds are first fermented and dried. The nibs are removed and roasted to develop the flavor further.
13. Cocoas may be divided into two main classes: natural-processed and Dutch-processed.
14. Chocolate has more fat in it than cocoa, and when substituting, 1 ounce unsweetened chocolate = 3 tablespoons cocoa plus 1 tablespoon fat.

I. TO SHOW SOME FACTORS WHICH AFFECT THE QUALITY OF COFFEE BEVERAGES

A. ELECTRIC PERCOLATED COFFEE

2 tablespoons regular grind coffee per cup of water

1. Put cold water in pot.
2. Put coffee in strainer, and adjust the strainer in the pot.
3. Cover and plug in the pot.
4. Pot will go through its cycle and percolate the coffee.
5. After percolator stops, allow the coffee to ripen 5 minutes before tasting.
6. Make pot at least 2/3 full.

B. AUTOMATIC DRIP COFFEE

1 tablespoon automatic drip-grind coffee per cup of water

1. Fill pot with desired amount of water.
2. Pour water into the top part of the coffee-maker.
3. Remove filter basket, add filter and desired amount of coffee.
4. Place filter basket into position.
5. Plug in coffee-maker and turn on.
6. After coffee-maker has gone through its cycle, allow coffee to ripen 5 minutes before tasting.
7. Serve within 30 minutes.

C. PREPARE DRIP COFFEE AND PERCOLATED COFFEE USING 2 TABLESPOONS OF COFFEE PER CUP OF WATER. RANK AND COMPARE COFFEES MADE BY THESE TWO METHODS FOR THE CHARACTERISTICS LISTED IN THE TABLE

TABLE FOR EVALUATION OF PERCOLATED AND DRIP COFFEE				
Method	Brownness	Clarity	Stimulating Aroma	Fresh, Mellow Taste*
Electric Percolated				
Automatic Drip				

*Absence of bitter or flat taste.

QUESTIONS

1. What were the differences between the ground coffees used for each method?

2. Which coffee had the most bitter flavor?

If so, why?

D. **INSTANT COMPARED WITH REGULAR COFFEE. PREPARE A SMALL POT OF MEDIUM STRENGTH INSTANT COFFEE FOLLOWING THE DIRECTIONS ON THE LABEL OF**

1. Regular instant
2. Decaffeinated instant

Compare instant coffee with that from the automatic drip grind. Rank for the characteristics listed in the table.

TABLE FOR EVALUATING INSTANT COFFEE VS. DRIP COFFEE			
Coffee	Stimulating Aroma	Strength	Fresh, Mellow Taste*
Automatic drip grind			
Regular instant			
Decaffeinated instant			

*Absence of bitter or flat taste.

QUESTIONS

1. How does the quality of freshly prepared coffee compare with that of instant coffee?

2. What effect, if any, does removal of the caffeine have upon the beverage?

II. TO SHOW SOME FACTORS WHICH AFFECT THE QUALITY OF TEA

A. STRENGTH OF TEA

Prepare small pots of tea using the following amounts of tea per cup of freshly boiling water:

1. 1/4 teaspoon
2. 1/2 teaspoon
3. 1 teaspoon
4. 2 teaspoons
5. 1 teabag

Pour boiling water over tea and allow the tea to steep 2-4 minutes. Pour half of the tea into cups for tasting hot and the other half over crushed ice in glasses for iced tea. Rank the teas for optimum strength in the table.

TABLE FOR EVALUATION OF EFFECT OF TEMPERATURE AND AMOUNT ON TEA STRENGTH		
Amount of Tea	Hot	Cold
1/4 teaspoon		
1/2 teaspoon		
1 teaspoon		
2 teaspoons		
1 teabag		

1. Account for the effects of the serving temperature on the amount of tea needed for optimum strength.

2. What amount of tea (in teaspoons) would be equivalent to 1 teabag?

B. KIND OF TEA

Prepare small pots of tea, using 1 teaspoon of tea per cup of water as follows:

1. Green tea
2. Oolong tea
3. Black tea

Rank green, oolong, and black tea for the characteristics listed in the table.

TABLE FOR EVALUATION OF DIFFERENT TEA VARIETIES				
Tea	Color	Aroma	Astringency	Briskness
Green				
Oolong				
Black				

QUESTION

1. What are the main differences between green, oolong, and black tea?

III. TO EVALUATE COCOA AND CHOCOLATE

A. CHOCOLATE

1/2 ounce unsweetened chocolate	2 cups milk
2 tablespoons sugar	1/4 teaspoon vanilla
1/2 cup water	

1. Combine water, chocolate, and sugar in a small saucepan. Heat to boiling with constant stirring. Continue boiling while stirring until a smooth paste forms. **CAUTION: DO NOT scorch mixture as it reaches consistency of paste**.
2. Add milk; heat to 200°F (94°C); add vanilla; serve.

B. COCOA

1 tablespoon cocoa	1 cup milk
1 tablespoon sugar	1/4 teaspoon vanilla
1/4 cup water	

1. Mix together cocoa and sugar in small saucepan; add water gradually; blend.
2. Heat to boiling with constant stirring. Continue boiling and stirring until smooth paste forms. **DO NOT allow mixture to scorch as it reaches consistency of paste.**
3. Add milk; heat to 200°F (94°C); add vanilla; serve.

TABLE FOR EVALUATION OF HOT CHOCOLATE			
Type	Color	Flavor	Body
Chocolate			
Cocoa			

QUESTIONS

1. What are the desired characteristics for a hot chocolate product?

2. Why was it important to keep the temperature below 200°F during preparation?

GENERAL QUESTIONS

1. What constituents in coffee contribute to the following:

   a. aroma?

   b. flavor?

   c. stimulating quality?

   d. color?

2. a. What type of deterioration takes place in roasted coffee?

   b. Under what conditions is deterioration retarded?

3.   What constituents in tea contribute to the following:

   a.   aroma?

   b.   appearance?

   c.   flavor?

   d.   stimulating quality?

4.   What food constituents are found in chocolate?

5.   What produces the reddish color in cocoa?

6.   What is the weight of the sections into which a pound of cooking chocolate is usually divided?

7.   How should chocolate be stored in the home?

8.   Why should cocoa powder and chocolate be cooked in making beverages?

9.   A recipe calls for 2 ounces of unsweetened chocolate. You are out of chocolate, but you do have cocoa. Can a substitution be made? If so, give directions.

LABORATORY 20

Sensory Evaluation
of Food

LABORATORY 20
SENSORY EVALUATION OF FOOD

When the quality of food is judged or evaluated by the senses (flavor, aroma, color, and texture), it is said to be sensory evaluation. Flavor of food is affected by temperature, color, and texture. This laboratory exercise will illustrate to the student how these different perceptions affect the identification and acceptability of a particular food item.

VOCABULARY

papilla   taste receptors
aftertaste   main taste sensations

I. TO STUDY THE EFFECT OF TEMPERATURE ON FLAVOR INTENSITY

The tongue is the main receptor which is effective in determining flavor of food. Temperature will also affect how flavor is perceived by the tongue.

Directions: Scoop vanilla ice cream into 3 separate cups. Taste the samples using the following temperatures:

-15°C (5°F): Sample #1
5°C (41°F): Sample #2
24°C (75°F): Sample #3

Rank the three samples by placing a check in the appropriate box. Remember to rinse your mouth between sampling.

TABLE FOR THE EVALUATION OF SWEETNESS INTENSITY			
Sweetness Intensity	Sample #1	Sample #2	Sample #3
Most sweet			
Moderately sweet			
Least sweet			

QUESTIONS

1. What affect did the temperature have on the perceived sweetness of the ice cream?

2. Where is the sweetness sensation located on the tongue?

3. What other sensory characteristic of ice cream is affected by sugar?

II. TO LEARN HOW COLOR AFFECTS FLAVOR

Color plays a central role in the evaluation of food. It not only influences the senses of taste and smell, but the acceptability of a food product.

Directions: Have the judge sit in a sensory panel booth and either be blindfolded or obscure the light with a piece of red cellophane paper. Present to the judge five fruit drinks that are different in color. Have the juice identified by flavor only since color will be obscured. Rinse between each sample. In the table provided, the judge will identify the juice in the order of presentation, and the reason for the selection.

TABLE FOR JUICE IDENTIFICATION	
Juice	Reason for Identifying
1.	
2.	
3.	
4.	
5.	

QUESTIONS

1. What influence does color or appearance have on

    a. taste perception?

    b. product acceptability?

III. TO DETERMINE HOW TEXTURE AFFECTS FOOD IDENTIFICATION

A food's textural attribute can also contribute to its identity and quality. Although a person's awareness of texture is not as apparent as their awareness of other food properties, when vast changes in texture are made, identification of foods can become difficult.

Directions: Present to the judges various foods that have been pureed (e.g., carrots, peas, prunes, etc.) or are naturally soft (e.g., cream of wheat, applesauce, cream cheese, etc.). The judge should be blindfolded or red cellophane installed over the light source of the testing booth so that color would not influence judgment. Rinse mouth between tasting. In the table provided, identify each food item in the order that they are presented, and the reason for your selection.

TABLE FOR IDENTIFICATION OF FOOD BY TEXTURE	
Food Item	Reason for Selection
1.	
2.	
3.	
4.	
5.	
6.	
7.	

1. What influence does texture have on acceptability and identification of food?

2. What role does sensory evaluation play in rating quality of food?

GLOSSARY

GLOSSARY

Acid:	(In terms of cooking) vinegar, lemon juice, or cream of tartar.
Amylopectin:	Highly branched chain fraction of starch.
Amylose:	Straight chain fraction of starch.
Antioxidant:	Substance that retards oxidative rancidity in fats by becoming oxidized itself and stopping a chain reaction.
Ascorbic Acid:	(Vitamin C) Available in powder and tablet form or in mixtures; may be used to prevent darkening of cut or peeled fruits such as apples, bananas, and peaches.
Bake:	To cook in an oven or oven-type appliance. Covered or uncovered containers may be used. When applied to meats in uncovered containers, method is generally called roasting.
Barbecue:	To roast slowly on a gridiron or spit, over coals, or under free flame or oven electric unit, usually basting with a highly seasoned sauce. Popularly applied to food cooked in or served with barbecue sauce.
Baste:	To moisten meat or other foods while cooking to add flavor and to prevent drying of the surface. The liquid is usually melted fat, meat drippings, fruit juice, sauce, or water.
Batter:	A mixture of flour and liquid, usually combined with other ingredients as in baked products. The mixture is of such consistency that it may be stirred with a spoon and is thin enough to pour or drop from a spoon.
Beat:	To make a mixture smooth by introducing air with a brisk, regular motion that lifts the mixture over and over, or with a rotary motion as with an egg beater or electric mixer.
Blanch:	(Precook) To preheat in boiling water or steam.
Bland:	Mild flavored, not stimulating to the taste; smooth, soft-textured.
Blend:	To mix thoroughly two or more ingredients.
Boil:	To cook water or a liquid consisting mostly of water in which bubbles rise continually and break on the surface. The boiling temperature of water at sea level is 212°F or 100°C.
Braise:	To cook meat or poultry slowly in a covered utensil in a small amount of liquid or in steam. (Meat may or may not be browned in a small amount of fat before braising.)
Bread:	To coat with crumbs of bread or other food; or to coat with crumbs, then with diluted slightly beaten egg or evaporated milk, and again with crumbs.
Brine:	A strong salt solution used in pickling, fermentation, and curing to inhibit growth of certain bacteria and provide flavor.
Broil:	To cook by direct heat.
Browning Reactions:	Darkening of some fruits when pared or cut due to oxidation of enzymes. Also, specific protein and sugar reactions.
Candied:	(1) Fruit, fruit peel, or ginger that is cooked in heavy syrup until plump and translucent, then drained and dried. The product is also known as crystallized fruit, fruit peel, or ginger. (2) Sweet potatoes or carrots, cooked in sugar or syrup. To candy a food is to cook it as described above.
Canner:	(Water Bath) A large, covered cooking utensil with side handles and jar holder. Capacity is designated by the volume of water that the canner will hold. The water capacity must assure a 2-4 inch coverage above the tops of the jars.
Caramelize:	To heat sugar or foods containing sugar until a brown color and characteristic flavor develop.
Carbohydrate:	Organic compounds containing carbon, hydrogen, and oxygen; simple sugars and polymers of simple sugars.
Carotenoids:	A variety of yellow to red pigments found in fruits and vegetables that are relatively stable to cooking methods.
Casserole:	A covered utensil in which food may be baked and served. It may have one or two handles. Size is stated in liquid measurements.
Cellulose:	A polysaccharide found in cell walls of plants, fruits, and vegetables that provides structural rigidity; can be softened by cooking but is not digested in the human alimentary tract.

Chlorophyll:	The green pigment found in vegetables that becomes olive-green when exposed to an acid cooking medium.
Chopped:	Cut into pieces with a knife or other sharp tool.
Coagulation:	The change from a fluid state to a thickened curd or clot due to denaturation of protein.
Colloidal Dispersion:	Combination of small particles and liquid in which the particles are too large to form a true solution and too small to form a coarse suspension; an example of a colloidal dispersion is gelatin and hot water.
Cream:	To soften a fat such as shortening or butter with a fork or other utensil, either before or while mixing with another food, usually sugar.
Creamed:	A term applied to foods that are either cooked in or served with a white sauce.
Crystallization:	Process of forming crystals that result from chemical elements solidifying with an orderly internal structure.
Curdle:	To effect a change from a smooth liquid to one in which clots float in a watery medium due to precipitation of protein by heat. Curdling may be observed in milk, cream soups and sauces, custards, and cheese dishes.
Cut:	To divide food materials with a knife or scissors.
Cut In:	To distribute solid fat in dry ingredients by chopping with knifes or pastry blender until finely divided.
Dash:	Less than 1/8 teaspoon of an ingredient, usually a spice.
Denaturation:	Changing of protein molecule, usually by the unfolding of chains, to a less soluble state.
Dextrinization:	Breakdown of starch molecules to dextrins by dry heat.
Dextrins:	Polysaccharides resulting from the partial hydrolysis of starch.
Dice:	To cut into small cubes.
Disperse:	To distribute or spread throughout some other substance.
Dough:	Mixture of flour and liquid, usually with other ingredients added. A dough is thick enough to knead or roll, as in making yeast bread and rolls, but is too stiff to stir or pour.
Dredge:	To cover or coat with flour or other fine substances such as bread crumbs or corn meal.
Dry Measure:	Measuring tool with capacity of 1 cup, 1/2 cup, 1/3 cup, or 1/4 cup (or 250 mL, 125 mL, and 50 mL). Capacity is based on the relation that one cup equals 16 level tablespoons.
Emulsification:	A process of breaking up large particles of liquids into smaller ones, which remain suspended in another liquid. Emulsification may be accomplished mechanically, as in the homogenization of ice cream mixtures; chemically with the use of acid and lecithin (from egg yolk) as in emulsification of oil for mayonnaise; or naturally, in body processes, as when bile salts emulsify fats during digestion.
Emulsify:	To make into an emulsion. When small drops of one liquid are finely dispersed (distributed) in another liquid, an emulsion is formed. The drops are held in suspension by an emulsifying agent, which surrounds each drop to form a coating.
Enzymatic Browning:	Discoloration found in cut fruit due to reaction of enzymes on exposure to oxygen.
Enzyme:	Protein substances that serve as organic catalysts in food effecting changes in color, texture, and flavor; inactivated by exposure to heat; activity retarded by refrigeration or freezing.
Fatty Acids:	Organic acids made up of chains of carbon atoms with a carboxyl group on one end; 3 fatty acids combine with glycerol to make a triglyceride.
Fermentation:	Chemical changes affected by yeast accompanied by production of alcohol and carbon dioxide.
Fill Weight:	Weight of fruit or vegetable in can as opposed to total weight including liquid.
Foam:	A type of colloidal dispersion in which bubbles of gas are surrounded by liquid; specific stability varies.
Fold:	To combine by using two motions, one which cuts vertically through the mixture, the other which turns it over by sliding the implement across the bottom of the mixing bowl.

Food Additives:	Substances added to a food during its preparation. Sometimes a substance is added to increase the concentration of a substance that may be naturally present in the food, such as the vitamins. Substances are added to protect the food against spoilage, enhance its flavor, improve its nutritive value, or give it some new property. Additives include chemical preservatives, buffers and neutralizers, nutrients, non-nutrient sweeteners, coloring agents, stabilizers, emulsifiers, and sequestrants. Some are generally recognized as safe; others are allowed for certain foods under certain conditions and in specified amounts. The Food and Drug Administration issues lists of permissible food additives.
Fricassee:	To cook by braising. Usually applied to fowl, rabbit, or veal cut into pieces.
Fry:	To cook in fat. Applied especially to (1) cooking in a small amount of fat, also called sauté or pan-fry; and (2) cooking in a deep layer of fat, also called deep-fat frying.
Gel:	A liquid in solid colloidal system that lacks the ability to flow; can be formed by gelatin, pectin, starch, soured milk, and egg.
Gelatinization:	The absorption of liquid by starch granules accompanied by swelling of the granules and thickening proportional to starch/liquid ratio. Process can proceed while cold, but heat is required to complete the physical change.
Grill:	To cook by direct heat. Also, a utensil or appliance used for such cooking.
Grind:	To reduce to particles by cutting or crushing.
Homogenize:	To break up into small particles of the same size. Homogenized milk has been passed through an apparatus to break the fat into such small globules that it will not rise to the top as cream. In homogenized shortening, air has been distributed evenly through the fat particles.
Hydration:	Process of absorbing water.
Hydrogenation:	A process in which hydrogen is combined chemically with an unsaturated compound, such as oil, to form solid or semi-solid fat.
Hydrolysis:	The process of splitting molecules into simpler components effected by acid and heat or by enzymes.
Immiscible:	Not capable of being mixed.
Ingredient Labeling:	System that requires food processors to list, on the label, ingredients (in descending order of weight) included in all manufactured items not covered by standards of identity.
International Unit (IU):	Measure of vitamin content, particularly in milk.
Inversion:	Chemical change that sucrose undergoes either when heated with acid or combined with the enzyme invertase in which the molecule is split into its components glucose and fructose.
Irradiation:	A process in which food is exposed to radiation. (See Radiation)
Jam:	A sweet preserve in which fruit and sugar are cooked together until a thick paste is formed and fruit becomes a homogeneous mass.
Jelly:	A gelled clear product that may be either sweet when made from fruit juice, or savory when made from meat stock.
Julienne:	Meats, fruits, or vegetables cut into slivers resembling matchsticks. Also a soup with thin strips of vegetables.
Kettle:	A covered or uncovered cooking utensil with a bail handle. Capacity is stated in liquid measurements.
Knead:	To manipulate with a pressing motion accompanied by folding and stretching.
Lactic Acid Bacteria:	Group of microorganisms which converts lactose to lactic acid; responsible for the souring of milk.
Leavening Agent:	Air, steam, or a microbiological or chemical agent capable of producing carbon dioxide when activated.
Legumes:	Seeds formed in pods such as peas and beans; the plant has the ability to fix nitrogen in the soil. Good source of protein.
Level Off:	To move the level edge of a knife or spatula across the top edge of a container, scraping away the excess material.
Liquid Measure:	Measuring tool with a capacity of one quart or less and equipped with a pouring lip for liquids. Capacities and subdivisions include quarts, pints, fluid ounces, or cups. Subdivisions are based on the relation that 1/2 pint equals 1 cup, 236.6 milliliters, or 8 fluid ounces.

Lukewarm:	Approximately 95°F or 35°C; tepid. Lukewarm liquids or foods sprinkled on the wrist will not feel warm.
Maillard Reaction:	Browning reaction involving combination of an amino group from a protein and an aldehyde group from a sugar that leads to the formation of many complex products.
Marinate:	To let food stand in a marinade which is a liquid, usually an oil-acid mixture such as French dressing.
Mask:	To cover completely. Usually applied to the use of mayonnaise or other thick sauce, but may also be applied to a flavor used as a mask or camouflage flavor.
Melt:	To liquify by use of heat.
Mince:	To cut or chop into very small pieces.
Mix:	To combine ingredients in any way that effects a distribution.
Monosodium Glutamate:	A chemical which is added to food to enhance flavor. Its effect on flavor depends on the kinds and amounts of other flavor factors in the food.
Nutrition Labeling:	Extensive nutritional information provided on labels of products making a nutritional claim or specifying nutrients added to the product.
Organic Foods:	Foods claimed to be grown without chemical fertilizers or pesticides. As there is no legal definition of this term, it is impossible to verify where used.
Osmotic Pressure:	Force that operates when fruit is simmered, directing the passage of water in or out of the cell, depending upon the surrounding liquid. Also occurs when fruits are sugared and allowed to stand or when a dressing has been held on a green salad for many minutes.
Oven Spring:	The rapid increase in volume of yeast bread during the first few minutes of baking.
Pan-Broil:	To cook, uncovered, on a hot surface, usually in a fry pan. Fat is poured off as it accumulates.
Pan-Fry:	To cook in a small amount of fat. (See Fry and Sauté)
Panning:	Method of cooking vegetables in their own juices in a tightly covered pan. A small amount of fat is used to moisten pan before juices escape.
Parboil:	To boil until partially cooked. Usually cooking is completed by another method.
Pare:	To cut off the outside covering.
Pasteurize:	To preserve food by heating and holding at a specific temperature for a specific length of time sufficient to destroy certain microorganisms and arrest fermentation. Applied to liquids such as milk and fruit juices. Temperatures used vary with foods but commonly range from 149°F to 180°F (60°C to 83°C).
Peel:	To strip off the outside covering.
Pickle:	Method of preserving food employing salt, brine, or vinegar.
Plasticity:	Ability to be molded or shaped.
Poach:	To cook in a hot liquid using precautions to retain shape. The temperature used varies with the food.
Polyphenols:	Organic compounds with an unsaturated ring and more than one -OH group; implicated in enzymatic browning in foods.
Polyunsaturated Fatty Acid:	Fatty acid that has two or more double bonds between carbon atoms.
Pome:	Fruit classification based on central core and presence of seeds; group includes apples, pears, and quinces.
Pot Roast:	A chunky piece of meat cooked by braising (see Braise).
Proofing:	The final rising period before baking for yeast doughs that have been molded.
Radiation:	The combined processes of emission, transmission, and absorption of radiant energy. Radiation is a method of food preservation in which small doses of ionizing radiation are applied to foods in order to prolong the shelf life of perishable foods, such as fresh seafood. Large doses of radiation (2 to 5 million rads) destroy microbial growth and sterilize the food. For food preservation applications, alpha and beta particles and gamma rays are radiations available. Quality of the finished product, as well as economic factors, have limited the commercial application of radiation as a means of food preservation.
Rancidity:	State of spoilage unique to fats in which the flavor and odor deteriorate due either to hydrolysis or oxidation.

Rehydration:	To soak, cook, or use other procedures with dehydrated foods to restore water lost during drying.
Render:	To free fat from animal tissues by heating at low temperatures.
Rennet:	Crude extract from calf stomach containing the enzyme rennin.
Retrogradation:	Tendency for gelatinized starch mixtures to form crystalline areas during storage (staling of baked products and starch pastes).
Roast:	To cook uncovered in hot air. Meat is usually roasted in an oven or over coals, ceramic briquettes, gas flame, or electric coils. The term also applies to foods such as corn or potatoes cooked in hot ashes, under coals, or on heated stones or metal.
Roux:	A thickening agent made by heating a blend of flour and fat. It may be white or brown and used in making gravies and sauces.
Saturated Fatty Acid:	Fatty acid contains no double bonds between its carbon atoms.
Saturated Solution:	Solution containing all the solute that it can dissolve at that temperature.
Sauté:	To brown or cook in a small amount of fat (see Fry).
Scald:	(1) To heat milk to just below the boiling point, when tiny bubbles form at edge; and (2) to dip certain foods in boiling water (see Blanch).
Scallop:	To bake foods (usually cut into pieces) with a sauce or other liquid. The food and sauce may be mixed together or arranged in alternate layers in a baking dish, with or without a topping of crumbs.
Sear:	To brown the surface of meat by a short application of intense heat.
Simmer:	To cook in a liquid just below the boiling point, at temperatures of 185°F to 210°F (85°C to 99°C). Bubbles form slowly and collapse below the surface.
Smoke Point:	Specific point for each fat at which it begins to smoke and emit irritating vapors when heated.
Solution:	A uniform liquid blend containing a solvent (liquid) and a solute (such as salt) dissolved in the liquid.
Sorbic Acid:	An antimycotic agent used in foods such as cheese to retard mold growth.
Steam:	To cook in steam with or without pressure. The steam may be applied directly to the food, as in a steamer or pressure cooker.
Steep:	To allow a substance to stand in liquid below the boiling point for the purpose of extracting flavor, color, or other qualities.
Sterilize:	To destroy microorganisms. Foods are most often sterilized at high temperatures with steam, hot air, or boiling liquid.
Stew:	To simmer food in a small amount of liquid.
Stir:	To mix food materials with a circular motion for the purpose of blending or securing uniform consistency.
Stir Fry:	Cooking method using tossing motions when cooking over high heat, particularly in oriental cuisines when a small amount of fat is used.
Supersaturated Solution:	Solution that has dissolved more solute or dispersed substance than it can normally hold at a particular temperature.
Suspension:	Combination of powder and liquid that remains combined only so long as agitation is continued. Solid will settle to bottom when undisturbed. Example: starch in cold water.
Syneresis:	Drainage of liquid from a gel system when cut or disturbed.
Texture:	Properties of food, including roughness, smoothness, graininess, creaminess, etc.
Textured Vegetable Protein:	Fabricated meats and meat extenders processed from soy beans providing excellent nutritive qualities and the potential for economy when sufficient volume can be utilized.
Toast:	To brown by means of dry heat.
Translucent:	Shining or glowing through; partly transparent.
Tuber:	Enlarged, fleshy portions of root systems growing underground that can reproduce when the "eyes" are planted (example: potatoes).
Viscosity:	A property of fluids that determines whether they flow readily or resist flow. A pure liquid at a given temperature and pressure has a definite viscosity, which usually increases with a decrease in temperature. Sugar syrups, for example, thicken as their temperatures decrease.

Whey:	Liquid portion of milk remaining after the curd, which is chiefly the protein casein, is precipitated.
Whip:	To rapidly beat such mixtures as gelatin dishes, eggs, and cream to incorporate air and increase volume.

APPENDIX A

Measuring Equivalents

Table of Equivalents

Pinch or dash	=	less than 1/8 teaspoon
3 teaspoons	=	1 tablespoon
2 tablespoons	=	1 fluid ounce
1 jigger	=	1 1/2 fluid ounces
4 tablespoons	=	1/4 cup
5 tablespoons + 1 teaspoon	=	1/3 cup
8 tablespoons	=	1/2 cup
10 tablespoons + 2 teaspoons	=	2/3 cup
12 tablespoons	=	3/4 cup
16 tablespoons	=	1 cup
1 cup	=	8 fluid ounces
2 cups	=	1 pint
2 pints	=	1 quart
4/5 quart	=	25.6 fluid ounces
1 quart	=	32 fluid ounces
4 quarts	=	1 gallon
2 gallons (dry measure)	=	1 peck
4 pecks	=	1 bushel

Some Fractional Measures

1/2 of 1/4 cup	=	2 tablespoons
1/2 of 1/3 cup	=	2 tablespoons + 2 teaspoons
1/2 of 1/2 cup	=	1/4 cup
1/2 of 2/3 cup	=	1/3 cup
1/2 of 3/4 cup	=	1/4 cup + 2 tablespoons
1/3 of 1/4 cup	=	1 tablespoon + 1 teaspoon
1/3 of 1/3 cup	=	1 tablespoon + 2 1/3 teaspoons
1/3 of 1/2 cup	=	2 tablespoons + 2 teaspoons
1/3 of 2/3 cup	=	3 tablespoons + 1 2/3 teaspoons
1/3 of 3/4 cup	=	1/4 cup

METRIC - U.S. EQUIVALENTS
(To second decimal place)

LENGTH		
1 millimeter*	=	0.04 inch
1 centimeter	=	0.39 inch
1 meter	=	39.37 inches
	=	1.09 yards
1 kilometer	=	0.62 statute mile

CAPACITY		
1 cubic centimeter	=	0.27 fluid dram
1 liter	=	1.06 liquid quarts

WEIGHT		
1 gram	=	0.04 ounce avoirdupois
1 kilogram	=	2.20 pounds avoirdupois
	=	1000 grams
1 metric ton	=	2204.62 pounds avoirdupois
	=	1.10 tons

EQUVALENTS OF THE COMMON CAPACITY UNITS USED IN THE KITCHEN

Units	Fluid Drams	Teaspoons	Table-spoons	Fluid Ounces	1/4 Cupful	Gills (1/2 Cupful)	Cupsful	Liquid Pints	Liquid Quarts	Milli-liters	Liters
1 fluid dram equals	1	3/4	1/4	1/8	1/16	1/32	1/64	1/128	1/256	3.7	0.004
1 teaspoon equals	1 1/3	1	1/3	1/6	1/12	1/24	1/48	1/64	1/192	4.9	0.005
1 tablespoon equals	4	3	1	1/2	1/4	1/8	1/16	1/32	1/64	15	0.015
1 fluid ounce equals	8	6	2	1	1/2	1/4	1/8	1/16	1/32	30	0.030
1/4 cupful equals	16	12	4	2	1	1/2	1/4	1/8	1/16	59	0.059
1 gill (1/2 cupful) equals	32	24	8	4	2	1	1/2	1/4	1/8	118	0.118
1 cupful equals	64	48	15	8	4	2	1	1/2	1/4	237	0.237
1 liquid pint equals	128	96	32	16	8	4	2	1	1/2	473	0.473
1 liquid quart equals	256	192	64	32	16	8	4	2	1	946	0.946
1 milliliter* equals	0.27	0.20	0.068	0.034	0.017	0.0084	0.0042	0.0021	0.0011	1	1/1000
1 liter equals	270	203	67.6	33.8	16.9	8.45	4.23	2.11	1.06	1000	1

*For all household purposes 1 milliliter may be considered as equal to 1 cubic centimeter.

APPENDIX B

Emergency
Substitutions

In a pinch, any of the following ingredient substitutions can be made successfully except in temperamental cakes, breads, cookies, or pastries.

LEAVENING

- 1 1/2 teaspoons phosphate or tartrate baking powder = 1 teaspoon double acting baking powder
- 1/4 teaspoon baking soda + 1/2 teaspoon cream of tartar = 1 teaspoon double acting baking powder
- 1/4 teaspoon baking soda + 1/2 cup sour milk = 1 teaspoon double acting baking powder in liquid mixtures; reduce recipe liquid content by 1/2 cup

THICKENING

- 1 tablespoon cornstarch = 2 tablespoons all-purpose flour
- 1 tablespoon potato flour = 2 tablespoons all-purpose flour
- 1 tablespoon arrowroot = 2 1/2 tablespoons all-purpose flour
- 2 teaspoons quick-cooking tapioca = 1 tablespoon all-purpose flour (use in soups only)

SWEETENING, FLAVORING

- 1 1/4 cups sugar + 1/3 cup liquid = 1 cup light corn syrup or honey
- 3 tablespoons cocoa + 1 tablespoon butter = 1 (1-ounce) square unsweetened chocolate
- 1/8 teaspoon cayenne pepper = 3-4 drops liquid hot red pepper seasoning

FLOUR

- 1 cup sifted all-purpose flour minus 2 tablespoons = 1 cup sifted cake flour
- 1 cup + 2 tablespoons sifted cake flour = 1 cup sifted all-purpose flour
- 1 cup sifted self-rising flour = 1 cup sifted all-purpose flour + 1 1/4 teaspoons baking powder and a pinch of salt

DAIRY

- 1/2 cup evaporated milk + 1/2 cup water = 1 cup whole milk
- 1 cup skim milk + 2 teaspoons melted butter = 1 cup whole milk
- 1 cup whole milk + 1 tablespoon lemon juice or white vinegar = 1 cup sour milk (let stand 5-10 minutes before using)
- 3/4 cup milk + 1/4 cup melted butter = 1 cup light cream

EGGS

- 2 egg yolks = 1 egg (for thickening sauces, custards)
- 2 egg yolks + 1 tablespoon cold water = 1 egg (for baking)
- 1 1/2 tablespoons stirred egg yolks = 1 egg yolk
- 2 tablespoons stirred egg whites = 1 egg white
- 3 tablespoons mixed broken yolks and whites = 1 medium-size egg

MISCELLANEOUS

- 1 cup boiling water + 1 bouillon cube or envelope instant broth mix = 1 cup broth
- 1 teaspoon beef extract blended with 1 cup boiling water = 1 cup beef broth
- 1 cup fine bread crumbs = 3/4 cup fine cracker crumbs
- 1/2 cup minced, plumped, pitted prunes or dates = 1/2 cup seedless raisins or dried currants
- 6 tablespoons mayonnaise blended with 2 tablespoons minced pickles or pickle relish = 1/2 cup tartar sauce

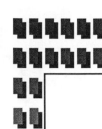

APPENDIX C

Retail Cuts of Meat

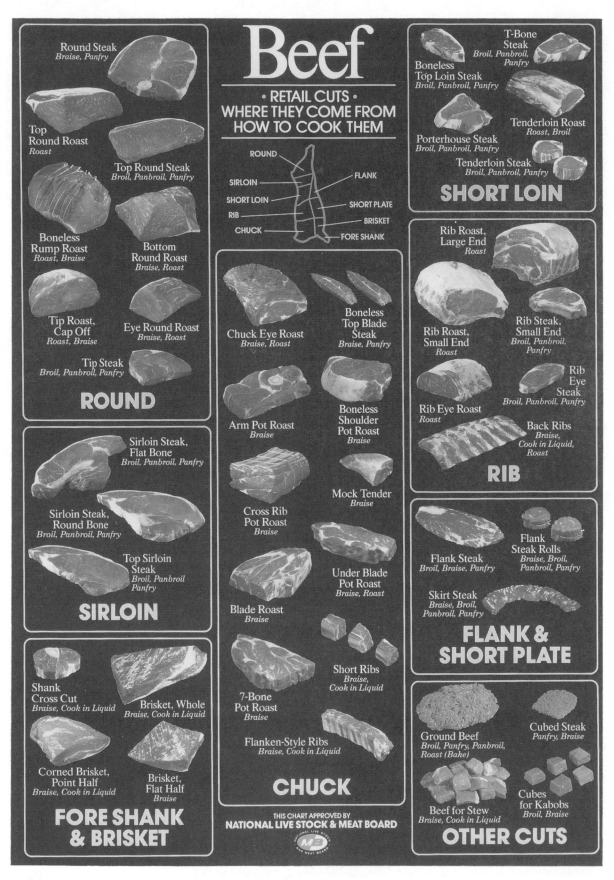

Beef

· RETAIL CUTS ·
WHERE THEY COME FROM
HOW TO COOK THEM

ROUND
SIRLOIN
SHORT LOIN
RIB
FLANK
SHORT PLATE
BRISKET
CHUCK
FORE SHANK

ROUND

Round Steak
Braise, Panfry

Top Round Roast
Roast

Top Round Steak
Broil, Panbroil, Panfry

Boneless Rump Roast
Roast, Braise

Bottom Round Roast
Braise, Roast

Tip Roast, Cap Off
Roast, Braise

Eye Round Roast
Braise, Roast

Tip Steak
Broil, Panbroil, Panfry

SIRLOIN

Sirloin Steak, Flat Bone
Broil, Panbroil, Panfry

Sirloin Steak, Round Bone
Broil, Panbroil, Panfry

Top Sirloin Steak
Broil, Panbroil Panfry

FORE SHANK & BRISKET

Shank Cross Cut
Braise, Cook in Liquid

Brisket, Whole
Braise, Cook in Liquid

Corned Brisket, Point Half
Braise, Cook in Liquid

Brisket, Flat Half
Braise

CHUCK

Chuck Eye Roast
Braise, Roast

Boneless Top Blade Steak
Braise, Panfry

Arm Pot Roast
Braise

Boneless Shoulder Pot Roast
Braise

Cross Rib Pot Roast
Braise

Mock Tender
Braise

Blade Roast
Braise

Under Blade Pot Roast
Braise, Roast

7-Bone Pot Roast
Braise

Short Ribs
Braise, Cook in Liquid

Flanken-Style Ribs
Braise, Cook in Liquid

SHORT LOIN

T-Bone Steak
Broil, Panbroil, Panfry

Boneless Top Loin Steak
Broil, Panbroil, Panfry

Porterhouse Steak
Broil, Panbroil, Panfry

Tenderloin Roast
Roast, Broil

Tenderloin Steak
Broil, Panbroil, Panfry

RIB

Rib Roast, Large End
Roast

Rib Roast, Small End
Roast

Rib Steak, Small End
Broil, Panbroil, Panfry

Rib Eye Roast
Roast

Rib Eye Steak
Broil, Panbroil, Panfry

Back Ribs
Braise, Cook in Liquid, Roast

FLANK & SHORT PLATE

Flank Steak
Broil, Braise, Panfry

Flank Steak Rolls
Braise, Broil, Panbroil, Panfry

Skirt Steak
Braise, Broil, Panbroil, Panfry

OTHER CUTS

Ground Beef
Broil, Panfry, Panbroil, Roast (Bake)

Cubed Steak
Panfry, Braise

Beef for Stew
Braise, Cook in Liquid

Cubes for Kabobs
Broil, Braise

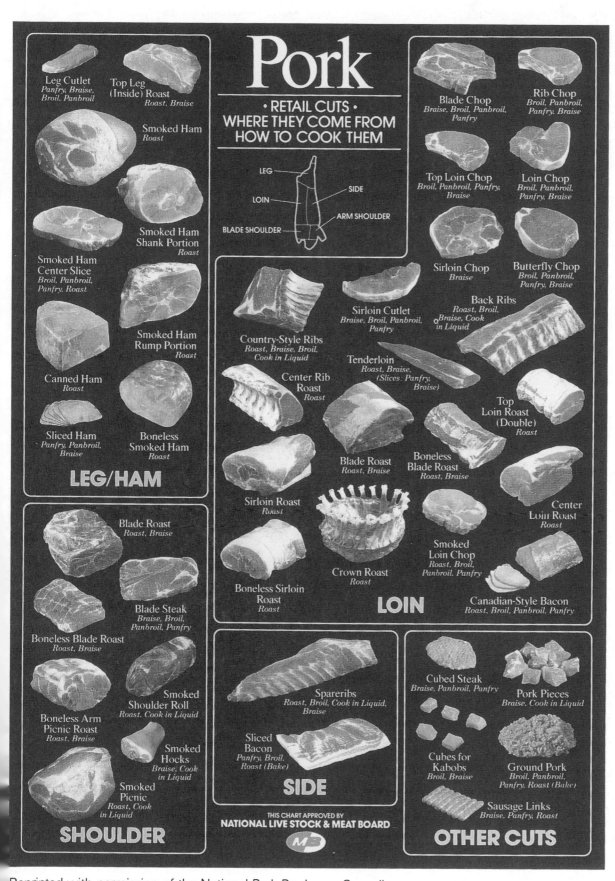

APPENDIX D

How To Identify Cuts of Meat by Bones

TYPE OF BONE	COMMON NAME	GENERAL COOKING METHOD
ARM Reprinted with the permission of General Mills, Inc. *Betty Crocker's Best Recipes for Meat and Vegetables*.	beef chuck arm steak beef chuck arm pot roast lamb shoulder arm chop lamb shoulder arm roast pork shoulder arm steak pork shoulder arm roast veal shoulder arm steak veal shoulder arm roast	braise, cook in liquid braise, cook in liquid braise, broil, panfry roast braise, panfry roast braise, panfry braise, roast
BLADE (center cuts) Reprinted with the permission of General Mills, Inc. *Betty Crocker's Best Recipes for Meat and Vegetables*.	beef chuck blade steak beef chuck blade pot roast lamb shoulder blade chop lamb shoulder blade roast pork shoulder blade steak pork shoulder blade Boston roast veal shoulder blade steak veal shoulder blade roast	braise, cook in liquid braise, cook in liquid braise, broil, panfry roast braise, broil, panfry braise, roast braise, panfry braise, roast
RIB (backbone and rib bone) Reprinted with the permission of General Mills, Inc. *Betty Crocker's Best Recipes for Meat and Vegetables*.	beef rib steak beef rib roast lamb rib chop lamb rib roast pork rib chop pork rib roast veal rib chop veal rib roast	broil, panfry roast broil, panfry roast braise, broil, panfry roast braise, panfry roast

TYPE OF BONE	COMMON NAME	GENERAL COOKING METHOD
LOIN (backbone; T-shape) Reprinted with the permission of General Mills, Inc. *Betty Crocker's Best Recipes for Meat and Vegetables.*	beef loin steak (T-bone, porterhouse) beef loin tenderloin roast or steak lamb loin chop lamb loin roast pork loin chop pork loin roast veal loin chop veal loin roast	broil, panfry roast, broil broil, panfry roast braise, broil, panfry roast braise, panfry roast, braise
HIP - Pin bone (near short loin) Reprinted with the permission of General Mills, Inc. *Betty Crocker's Best Recipes for Meat and Vegetables.*	beef sirloin steak beef loin tenderloin roast or steak	broil, panfry roast, broil
Flat bone (center cut) Reprinted with the permission of General Mills, Inc. *Betty Crocker's Best Recipes for Meat and Vegetables.*	lamb sirloin chop lamb leg roast pork sirloin chop pork sirloin roast	broil, panfry roast braise, broil, panfry roast
Wedge bone (near round) Reprinted with the permission of General Mills, Inc. *Betty Crocker's Best Recipes for Meat and Vegetables.*	veal sirloin steak veal leg sirloin roast	braise, panfry roast

TYPE OF BONE	COMMON NAME	GENERAL COOKING METHOD
LEG (leg or round bone) Reprinted with the permission of General Mills, Inc. *Betty Crocker's Best Recipes for Meat and Vegetables*.	beef round steak beef rump roast lamb leg steak lamb leg roast pork leg (ham) steak pork leg roast (fresh or smoked) veal leg round steak veal leg roast	braise, panfry braise, roast broil, panfry roast braise, broil, panfry roast braise, panfry braise, roast
BREAST (breast and rib) Reprinted with the permission of General Mills, Inc. *Betty Crocker's Best Recipes for Meat and Vegetables*.	beef brisket (fresh or corned) beef plate short rib lamb breast lamb breast riblet pork bacon (side pork) pork sparerib veal breast veal breast riblet	braise, cook in liquid braise, cook in liquid roast, braise braise, cook in liquid broil, panfry, bake roast, braise, cook in liquid roast, braise braise, cook in liquid

APPENDIX E

Sanitation in the Kitchen

SANITATION IN THE KITCHEN

The objective is to remove food particles as well as other soil, and to control bacteria. All equipment and utensils must be expected to contain food spoilage bacteria as well as pathogens (disease causing bacteria). Proper cleaning removes soil. Sanitizing reduces the bacterial load to a safe level. Proper water temperature and proper amounts of cleaning compound must be used for an effectual job. It is essential to use a cleaning compound or detergent along with a brush (mechanical or hand activated) to loosen food remnants. A thorough rinsing must follow in order to sanitize the surfaces to achieve the desired bacterial action.

Sanitation Rules that should be followed:

1. All raw fruit and vegetables must be washed before being cooked or served.
2. Cold food should be kept cold and hot foods should be kept hot.
3. Get food hot as quickly as possible and keep it hot; above 140°F.
4. Get food cold as quickly as possible and keep it cold; 40°F or below.
5. Do not expose foods to the Danger Zone (40°F to 140°F) for more than 2 hours.
6. Separate surfaces should be used for the cutting, cubing and portioning of raw meats and poultry, and for cooked food items.
7. Each time a person has had contact with uncooked items, which may be suspected of carrying pathogens, he or she must wash his or her hands before handling cooked items.
8. Always sanitize your work area before beginning any type of food preparation. Use a solution of bleach and water.
9. If in doubt about the safety or quality of the food, throw it out.
10. Keep food covered as much as possible; use clean utensils.

Washing Dishes

Hand dishwashing should follow the following directions:

1. Fill sink or pan with hot water (120°F [49°C] or above). Add enough detergent to make light suds.
2. Rinse dishes and utensils in clean hot water.
3. Avoid towel drying your dishes, glasses or utensils.
4. Use any recommended soap or detergent that will be adequate in cleaning as well as sanitizing.

Machine Dishwashing

1. Remove all food particles from dishes, using either a scraper or the rinse water power arm.
2. Pre-rinse dishes at 80°F. Wash at 140°F and rinse at 180°F. Avoid toweling dishes.
3. Store dishes in a clean, dry, enclosed storage area. Invert cups and glasses.
4. Use any recommended soap or detergent that will be adequate in cleaning as well as sanitizing.

APPENDIX F

Safe Food Storage

A. Safe Storage in Refrigerator

CANNED GOODS	
Fruit	5-7 days
Jams and Jellies	6 months
Mayonnaise	1-2 months
Meats	1-2 days
Pickles	2-3 months
Vegetables	2-3 days
MEATS	
Fresh beef, lamb, pork, and veal:	
Roasts	2-4 days
Steaks, chops	3 days
Ribs	2 days
Stew meat	2 days
Ground meat	1-2 days
Processed meats, after package is opened:	
Ham, whole and half	7 days
Bacon	5-7 days
Frankfurters	4-5 days
Luncheon meats, sliced	3 days
Fresh fish	1-2 days
Poultry	1-2 days
DAIRY	
Butter and margarine	1 month
Buttermilk	1-2 weeks
Cheese (opened):	
Hard, Swiss, Cheddar	3-4 weeks
Parmesan, grated	1 year
Soft, cream, Neufchatel	2 weeks
Cottage	5-7 days or package date
Eggs	1 month
Half-and-Half	7-10 days
Milk: Whole and skim	1 week
Sour cream	3-4 weeks
Whipping cream	10 days

B. Safe Storage In Pantry

CANNED GOODS	
Fruit	1 year
Vegetables	1 year
Soup	1 year
Meat, fish, and poultry	1 year
PACKAGED MIXES	
Cake mix	1 year
Casserole mix	18 months
Frosting mix	8 months
Pancake mix	6 months
STAPLES	
Baking powder and soda	1 year
Breakfast Cereal:	
Ready-to-Eat	check package date
Uncooked	1 year
Coffee (opened and refrigerated)	6-8 months
Cornmeal: Regular and self-rising	10 months
Dried beans and peas	18 months
Flour:	
All-purpose	10-15 months
Whole wheat (refrigerated)	3 months
Grits:	
Regular	10 months
Instant, flavored	9 months
Milk: Evaporated and sweetened condensed	1 year
Pasta	10-15 months
Peanut butter	6 months
Salt, pepper, sugar	18 months
Shortening	8 months
Spices:	
Ground	6 months
Whole (discard if aroma fades)	1 year
Tea bags	1 year
Vegetable oil	3 months
Worcestershire sauce	2 years

C. Safe Storage in Freezer

BAKED GOODS	
Bread	3 months
Cakes	3-5 months
Cookies	6 months
Pies and pastry	2 months
DAIRY	
Butter	6 months
Cheese	4 months
Ice Cream	1-3 months
Eggs:	
White	6 months
Yolk	8 months
FISH AND SHELLFISH	
Fat fish	3 months
Lean fish	6 months
Shellfish	3 months
POULTRY	
Chicken, whole	3-6 months
Chicken, pieces	3 months
Chicken, cooked	1 month
Turkey	6 months
MEAT	
Beef	6-12 months
Pork	3-6 months
Lamb	6-9 months
Veal	6-9 months
Ground meats	3-4 months
Ham	1-2 months
Bacon	1 month
Frankfurters	1 month
Sausage	2 months
Variety meats	3-4 months
Leftover cooked meat	3 months
VEGETABLES AND FRUITS	
Vegetables, commercially frozen	8 months
Vegetables, home frozen	12 months
Fruits, commercially frozen	12 months
Fruits, home frozen	12 months

APPENDIX G

Care and Cleaning of Small Appliances

BLENDERS

1. Unplug; remove blender jar; remove all parts and place in **hot soapy water**. Use a dish cloth to wash parts. Rinse in hot water and drain.
2. Use a damp (not wet) cloth to wipe blender base. Wrap cord around top.
3. When parts are dry, **do not assemble**; blades need to air dry longer.
4. Place base and jar on cart.

HAND MIXERS

1. Unplug; remove beaters and place in hot soapy water. Wash thoroughly. Rinse in hot water and drain.
2. Use a damp (not wet) cloth to wipe mixer. Wrap cord around.
3. When beaters are dry, replace in mixer. Return to cart.

STAND MIXERS

1. Unplug; remove beater and place in **hot soapy water**.
2. Wash thoroughly and rinse in hot water; drain.
3. Use a damp (not wet) cloth to wipe mixer. Wrap cord around neck.
4. Replace clean bowl and place beater in bowl.

SIFTERS - DO NOT WET!!!

1. Tap gently over trash can to remove excess flour.
2. Use a dry cloth or paper towel to wipe all traces of flour.
3. Return to cart.

DEEP FAT FRYERS

1. Unplug; cover; leave on counter.
2. Label lid with use of the oil.